GETTING PERSONAL

Stories of Life with Tourette Syndrome

GETTING PERSONAL
Stories of Life with Tourette Syndrome

■ ■ ■

edited by
Michael G. DeFilippo

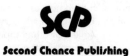

Second Chance Publishing
Lebanon, Tennessee
www.secondchancepublishing.com
info@secondchancepublishing.com

■ ■ ■

For my son, Andrew
You are my proudest moment
and my greatest accomplishment.

■ ■ ■

"To do nothing is in every man's power."

—Samuel Johnson

ACKNOWLEDGEMENTS

As a reader of books, I must admit that I rarely took the time to read acknowledgments. I suppose it was more anticipating reading the story than flagrant disregard for an author's thanks. However, after having worked on this project, I now read the acknowledgements before moving on to the story. I ask all of you to please read my expressions of gratitude. I have learned that these folks to whom I give thanks are the single, most important part of this, or any book. Please help me to thank them all for their unselfish contributions to this project and to my life.

All of the stories in this book were written by individuals who have, in some way, had their lives touched by this disorder. I requested these stories, and much to my surprise, so many brave folks responded. All of these individuals did not know me, yet they were willing to share their personal lives with me and with you. I thank each and every one of them from the bottom of my heart for having the courage to expose their darkest secrets. For some of us, writing a story this personal was one of the hardest things we have ever done.

For the few individuals who requested that I withhold your identities, I offer a very special thank you, because you have given me the highest honor I could receive: you have trusted me with your lives.

I consider myself fortunate in that I have made a friend for life in each and every person who contributed to this book. Our lives intersected at a place where few lives do: the crossroads of familiarity and respect. For these gifts I am eternally grateful.

I thank all of the contributors to this book: Rachel Arsenault, Teri Bernhardt, Greg Blackburn, Arthella Carpenter, Brad Cohen, Robert Cook, Eric Daily, Vernon Frazer, Shawna Rae Fross, Jonathan Gennick, Robert Jones*, Eileen Kelly*, Deborah Lynch, Leonard William Misner, Angela C. Reinheimer, Marlene Remley, Kathryn A. Taubert, Colleen Wang, Allison Faith Zalaman, Patti*, and Vicki*.

Many heartfelt thanks to Martin H. Wagner, M.D., for a diagnosis that ended thirty-three years of self-doubt.

Thank you, Andrew K. Stone, for letting me pick your brain about all matters relating to books; thanks to Vernon Frazer, for all of your invaluable advice; and special thanks to Leonard William Misner for your help with this book.

Many thanks to B. Duncan McKinlay, Ph.D., for his most touching foreword.

Thanks to Joanne Cohen, LICSW, B. Duncan McKinlay, Ph.D, Sheila Rogers, Rosie Wartecker, and Michael Wolff for taking time out of your busy schedules to read the manuscript and for your kind words.

Thanks to Gretchen Schuler for designing the interior layout and the book cover. You are a gem.

To my sister, Gina DeFilippo, I love you so much for helping to raise me after Mom and Dad crossed over. You have been an inspiration and I hope that someday I will have your strength. Thanks also for your photographic skills. Wendy Gray, you have been like a sister to me, always providing and never judging. I love you dearly.

To my Godparents, John and Helen Guercio, thank you so much for being there whenever I need you.

To my son, Andrew, thank you for showing me what only you can—the world through a child's eyes. I love you more than life itself.

To my ex-wife, Kathleen, if everyone understood Tourette syndrome the way that you do, this book would not be necessary.

To Dave and Amy Loewy, Regina Cannizzaro, Dean Remel, Denise Marks, Connie and Mickey Eakes, Angel Loupe, Misty Harper, Lisa Blue, Mary Bennett, Dee Odle, Beverly Shrum, Sonja Loeffler, Tammy Burney, and Donna West. Thanks for being my friends.

Many thanks to Cecelia Cox, President of the Tourette Syndrome Association of Tennessee, for teaching me much of what I know about Tourette syndrome.

Thanks to Laura Paley for giving me a chance, albeit brief, to see what my life could be like without Tourette syndrome.

To everyone at Rademacher's Chop House, the best restaurant in middle Tennessee! Thanks for your patience and for making me feel like part of your family. It has been great working with all of you.

Thanks to Elizabeth Rainwater for her editorial work on the introduction, Greg Blackburn's *The Will to Overcome*, Kathryn Taubert's *The Business of Living*, and my story, *Up Close and Personal*, and to Jenny Frances Carr for editing *My Precious Gifts* by Arthella Carpenter.

Lastly, I would like to thank you, the reader, for giving all of us an audience. I hope that you find a little bit of yourself in our stories, or recognize someone you know who may have had similar experiences.

An asterisk next to a contributor's name indicates that that contributor wishes to remain anonymous.

PREFACE

Unbeknownst to me, this project started in 1965 when at the age of seven, I began ticcing during a television commercial for a food product. Subsequently, every time I heard this product's jingle, I would jerk my head downward. I know this seems like strange behavior, but then again, most Tourettic tics appear strange when observed by others.

The symptoms and severity of Tourette syndrome vary greatly, as do the stories in this book. This serves my purpose well: to present Tourette's as a condition that is complex in nature and not easily defined. Due to sensationalism in the media, Tourette syndrome is still largely thought of as the "cursing disease." I hope that the stories in this book will help to dispel this longstanding myth.

This book is meant to educate. There are thousands of teachers and doctors, aunts and uncles, sisters and brothers, and mothers and fathers who are affected by or will be affected by Tourette syndrome. I want to reach out to all of these groups and attempt to show, through the stories in this book, what Tourette syndrome is and what it isn't. I want the public to understand what we experience as a result of our close relationship with this disorder.

Because there are a host of books available that present the medical side of Tourette syndrome, which is so dynamic, I did not want to write another book that leaves so much unexplained. I decided that the best way to do this was to let those of us with Tourette syndrome tell our stories. I let these folks tell their stories without interruption from me. Changes I have made were to clarify and enhance, not to correct and critique. The voices are theirs, the emotions are theirs, and the personalities are theirs. Any mistakes, typographical errors, misspellings, or inconsistencies are mine, and mine alone.

Where contributors have supplied details about medications, I have included this information so others can see examples of particular medications at work. I have taken the liberty, with the contributors' permission, to remove dosage amounts; however, the drug name and frequency of dosage has been retained. To avoid confusion, I have included the brand name of the drug, followed by the generic name in parentheses. These medications are specific to the individuals in this book, and are in no way meant to be indicative of your experience with the same drugs or with the helpfulness or harmfulness of any particular drug. Everyone has different reactions and each medication affects an individual in a unique way. What may not work for one person may be a Godsend for the next. Please consult your doctor before you begin any drug therapy.

This book has been a labor of love for the past two years and I am honored that you are holding it in your hands.

Michael G. DeFilippo
Lebanon, Tennessee
September, 2002

FOREWORD

I was extraordinarily flattered when Michael approached me to write the foreword for this book, so I immediately set to work mentally sketching the perfect ("just right") outline. In doing so, I contemplated the road my life has taken over the past decade since my own diagnosis. I mused about the lessons I had initially resisted, rejected, despised and endured, and have ultimately accepted, appreciated and valued, and wondered which kernels would be most valuable to impart upon you, the reader. I waxed philosophic on issues of attitude, the meaning of disorder and wellness, the interplay of one person's rights against another's, and competing opinions on treatment and symptom accountability. I waded through all of my own writings, searching for nuggets of profoundness to share. Then it occurred to me that perhaps I should actually read the book....

What a relief to find that I need not say anything, for contained within is a staggering amount of wisdom all put much more elegantly than I could ever hope to. As I moved from one vignette to the next I learned, and my sense of awe increased along with my humility.

Greg's discovery that love, faith, and a diagnosis wields infinitely more influence than any symptom-masking medication could ever hope to muster is similar to Deborah's observation that finding the right environment for who you are is not only great medicine, but it has substantially fewer side-effects. These two views are nicely countered by Eileen's "prescription" to her increased self-comfort and success in a world that does not always fit well with certain symptoms. Finally, Vicki shows us how *treatment* does not have to be synonymous with *drug* at all.

Kathryn delivers a most poignant message that unconditional acceptance and tenacity makes even an "It" bearable, and Patti and Arthella show us that there are few forces in the universe more unconditional and tenacious than the love of a mother. Rachel exemplifies the benefits of "coming clean" to your friends, and Allison delineates a phenomenal way in which to do so. Both Angela and Teri assure that the education of others brings good strategies, better times, and support that can both astound you in its quantity and stir you in its quality, while Shawna champions self-acceptance as the door that opens to a better way of living. And while Eric voices gratitude to the media for giving his differences a name, Marlene and Colleen picked their answers from the family tree and Robert ponders possible environmental causes and/or triggers for Tourette's.

Each story is different—each person is different. But each individual contained within has a valuable message. These are sages offering you personal revelations and perceptions both astute and far beyond their years. They are husbands and boyfriends, wives and girlfriends, mothers, fathers, children, and pillars of their communities. In one disclosure you may see enormous resilience despite daunting circumstances. In another you may see a child who takes full advantage of his or her Tourette-amplified talents, having grown up educated in and comfortable with his or her differences. They've sweated, strained, huffed and puffed in life's gymnasium; their tears and perseverance mean that others can now admire the bulging muscles labeled musician (Vernon), distinguished educator (Brad), poet (Robert), scholar (Leonard), computer programmer (Jonathan), and writer (Michael) that grace and sculpt their attractive frames.

my name is duncan. i have tourette syndrome. i have rather pronounced motor and phonic symptoms. so far, i have chronic neck and back problems, severe headaches, intermittent vocal cord strain, and a danger of eye damage as a result. i have people react to me in all manners of offensiveness every day. i have always had difficulty in relationships with my parents, my sister, and partners i've dated, in part due to the impulsivity, obsessive compulsiveness, explosivity, and social skills deficits i also contend with. i have faced and been forced to swallow discrimination from universities, employers, and internship sites to which i've applied over the years, and at 28, i feel much, much older than i actually am.

My name is Dr. McKinlay. I have a Ph.D. in Psychology. I have devised, successfully tested, and published a comprehensive neuropsychobiological model of how tics are formed in the brain. I have a job as a Psychologist that will evolve from a supervised position to one of fully registered autonomous practice. I have an international presentation and consultation business, a thriving Web site, two syndicated columns, an award-winning documentary film about me, many wonderful friends and loving families in my life, a musical inclination that has led me to both drumming and singing, a great sense of humour, the ability to think, speak, comprehend and sense, two arms, two legs, and a good heart.

My name is Dr. Bruce Duncan McKinlay. I have *power*. While *all* of the above statements about me are true, this one quality is of the utmost importance. I have an ability that not a single other entity on the planet can usurp from me. I, and I alone, decide each morning when I wake up which description above will be how *I* live my life. This freedom is staggering in its enormity—at once it hits you that symptoms, parents, teachers, bullies, bosses, or the partners that never understood you are not the biggest issues at all. *You are.* Decide for yourself—truly *believe and trust*—that you are okay, and your enslavement ends. Then you, too, will find that your own second paragraph starts to develop.

It is an honour and a privilege to find myself associated in print with the individuals you are about to meet. If, in the midst of working your way through this book, you find yourself at times forgetting that these are the words of the disordered, then you are starting to get it. If, as you finish the volume, it occurs to you that there is not a single victim of Tourette syndrome to be found within these pages, well, then give yourself a pat on the back because you really got it. Welcome to the club, my friend. Enjoy.

B. Duncan McKinlay, Ph.D.,
www.lifesatwitch.com

CONTENTS

GETTING PERSONAL

Stories of Life with Tourette Syndrome

INTRODUCTION

Michael G. DeFilippo

Amidst the muffled conversations of a quiet, softly lit restaurant, a man raises his voice. "Stop twitching! You're embarrassing me!" he snaps at a little boy. Diners near them turn puzzled stares their way. More quietly, but still irritated, the man finishes, "Every week it's some new habit with you!" The seven-year old squirms in his seat and looks down at a water circle on the tablecloth. He is trying for his very best table manners. The boy's right wrist jerks again, as if it were the wrist of a marionette, yanked from above by a string. This time the movement is so severe that kernels of corn fly from his fork through the air and become yellow dots on the brown-carpeted floor. This time they both look at the tablecloth and pretend not to notice.

■ ■ ■

"Hey, Twitchy!" yells the classroom bully, jerking his chin up, then down, and then to the right. He is mimicking a teenager sitting three rows away, and he is making sure that every student occupying a desk within view will see his show. "What's the matter? You retarded or something?" The classroom fills with chuckles and giggles, and then with laughter. A thirteen-year-old head, object of the derision, jerks again. Another string is pulled, and the shoulder twitches violently into the chair back. He mumbles something about being nervous about the quiz. More laughter. Clenching his teeth, the student waits. His worry about the upcoming quiz is blanketed by his desperation for the teacher to appear, for the bell to ring, and for the 50 minutes of peace that will follow.

■ ■ ■

Two college students cross a campus quadrangle on their way to a physics class, where a mid-term exam awaits them. "Whatcha got on your shoe?" asks the taller of the two. "Oh, nuthin', just a foot itch and no time to stop and scratch," answers the student on the left. He has intentionally positioned himself to the left of his walking partner, hoping to shield the involuntary movements from notice. As they continue their trek, his left knee bends again and brings his foot up, and his left hand reaches behind him to slap the left side of his shoe heel. His foot then slams the ground, yet he never breaks his stride. The companion is curious, but makes no further query. Eight more times, before they reach their destination, the shorter man slaps his raised left heel, jerked up by the puppeteer, and stomps the ground with his left foot, in an effort to simulate a normal walk.

■ ■ ■

In a kid-theme restaurant, a father emits a barely audible grunt and tightens his lip muscles around his mouth to mute the sounds that want to get out. His little boy, about three years old, watches. The sound is followed by a subtle but noticeable head jerk, and the father bounces ever so slightly on his booth bench. As the man calculates the gratuity for the guest check, he notices his son begin to sway his head from side to side, slowly at first, and then with more force. The boy stops and smiles his delighted silly-smile when he notices his father is watching. The man looks at his son with wonder, returns the glee with his own silly-smile, and reaches for his wallet. Is the toddler just mimicking his daddy? Or has his own puppeteer picked up his strings and begun to work? Although the father may not always know what to do, he is glad that he knows what *not* to do. He gathers his son into his arms, and they stop to laugh together at the huge balloon clown near the door.

■ ■ ■

These four vignettes span thirty-six years of one life. The little boy whose wrist jerks, the teenager whose head snaps up, down, and sideways, the young man whose hand slaps his up-drawn heel, and the father who remembers not to watch his son too closely. They are all me.

Tourette syndrome is the puppet-master. This highly mis-understood and misrepresented disorder pulls the strings that invoke this strange behavior we call "tics."

These are not isolated incidents, but snapshots of a life lived with Tourette syndrome. They have occurred hundreds, if not thousands of times over the course of my life. But these experiences are not mine alone. They are shared by many others with Tourette syndrome.

This book of first-person accounts is intended to allow you, the reader, to walk along with many people who have lived their entire lives in a state of "trying not to tic," knowing as no one else can that there is nothing they can do to prevent it. The feelings of embarrassment, shame, disgrace, and deceit that go along with Tourette syndrome are ruthless in their con-sistency and indescribable in their depth. All of these feelings emanate from the lack of knowledge, understanding, and acceptance by a world that frames those who are different.

More than just an intent to invoke empathy with suffering, however, what will come as you read these stories, will be a sense of warmth—a comfort with your own discoveries to be found in them. Compassion is not just empathy or sympathy. It is understanding that, for people who are different, all it takes to ameliorate the damaging emotions that so often accompany their differences is simple acceptance. If one college friend on one college campus can brighten a day with the ability to observe, know, and be honestly sensitive to his friend's "oddness," it follows that a world full of such friends, known and unknown, can make the fright of being teased and ostracized disappear. These stories are not just for those whose lives are affected by Tourette syndrome. They are for all—to entertain, inform, educate, and bring a sense of acceptance— for only when it is as "okay" to have Tourettic tics as it is to have a limp from a football injury, will the puppet master's enslavement end.

WHAT IS TOURETTE SYNDROME?

Michael G. DeFilippo

Tourette syndrome (TS) is difficult to pin down and more difficult to characterize by one set of criteria. I have spent many hours researching the disorder and interviewing many individuals, both for the book and to add to my knowledge. Although I have TS, I am constantly amazed at how much I learn day to day, both about myself and about the disorder.

Definition

TS is an inherited, neurobiological disorder characterized by repeated physical movements and vocalizations called tics.

The symptoms of TS typically appear before the age of eighteen, more commonly before the age of ten. Given the genetic predisposition, males are three to four times more likely to exhibit symptoms than are females.

Biologically, TS is caused by an imbalance in the brain's neurotransmitters, the chemicals that transport messages between nerve cells. Dopamine, the chemical that controls movement, has long been known to be involved with TS. Serotonin, which controls mood, hunger, aggressiveness, sleep, and is linked to obsessive-compulsive disorder, and norepinephrine, which controls heart rate and blood pressure, have recently been associated with TS. In more current research, brain scans have shown abnormalities in the size and functioning of certain parts of the brain in people with TS. Environmental factors, such as illness and infection, can possibly be associated with the onset of TS.

The true incidence of TS worldwide is not known because no formal epidemiology has been done. Since the disorder is so complex and no diagnostic medical test exists, it depends on who you consult as to what the answer is. In my research I have seen a range anywhere from 1 in 2000 to 1 in 100.

Types of Tics

The physical movements are called motor tics, and the vocalizations are referred to as vocal tics. Each group can be further divided into two types of tics, simple and complex.

Simple motor tics include eye blinking, facial grimacing, head jerking, abdominal contractions, and shoulder-shrugging. Examples of complex motor tics are licking, spitting, squatting, jumping, touching and smelling things, copropraxia, echopraxia, and palipraxia.

Copropraxia involves involuntary obscene or inappropriate gestures. *Echopraxia* is the imitation of other people's actions. *Palipraxia* is a repetitive action, as when an individual repeatedly flips a light switch on and off.

Vocalizations can take many forms. Simple vocal tics include throat clearing, sniffing, snorting, and grunting, and complex vocal tics are coprolalia, echolalia, and palilalia.

Coprolalia is when an individual involuntarily utters or shouts obscenities or socially inappropriate epithets. Coprolalia isn't defined by only these two types of outbursts; anything that is inappropriate to a given situation may also be uttered. These outbursts are not intentional. (This symptom occurs in roughly ten percent of the TS population, and in recent years has shown a decline that I believe is the result of the greater number of cases of TS in which coprolalia does not appear that are being diagnosed each year.) *Echolalia* is the imitation of other people's speech, and is a shared trait with some Autistic individuals. *Palilalia* involves the repetition of one's last phrase, sentence, word, or syllable.

No two individuals affected by TS necessarily have the same tics. Tics also tend to wax and wane throughout one's life. At some points the tics can be frequent and severe, and at other times they can virtually disappear. This makes it difficult to determine if a reduction in tics is due to a particular medication or the waning of symptoms.

An important point that requires discussion is the use of the term *involuntary* when defining tics. When I began researching TS early in 1998, I dismissed the possibility of my having the disorder because tics were described as *involuntary movements*. When I hear the term involuntary, I imagine a muscle spasm. It happens all by itself and there is nothing you can do to stop it; eventually, it goes away. I did not believe that my tics were reflexive. I knew I was doing it. I was making them happen. I could even control them for a time, but not indefinitely. Not until I came across the phrase *uncontrollable urge* did I make the connection between my behavior and TS. This phrase put it in perspective for me.

What Are the Diagnostic Criteria for Tourette Syndrome?

According to the Diagnostic and Statistical Manual of Mental Disorders (DSMV-IV), the criteria for a diagnosis of TS are as follows:

1. Both multiple motor and one or more vocal tics have

been present at some time during the illness, although not necessarily at the same time.

2. The tics occur many times a day (usually in bouts), nearly every day, or intermittently throughout a period of more than one year, and during this period there was never a tic-free period of more than three consecutive months.

3. The disturbance causes marked distress or significant impairment in social, occupational, or other important areas of functioning.

4. The onset is before age 18.

5. The disturbance is not due to the direct physiological effects of a substance or a general medical condition.

Why Is Tourette Syndrome So Difficult to Diagnose?

Many children, and for that matter, many adults, are not being diagnosed with TS because its symptoms are misunderstood or not known at all. To further complicate matters, the symptoms that are presented in the media via television and movies are exaggerated and sensationalized, leading to more confusion. A child in a classroom who is flipping his hair out of his eyes, blinking rapidly, tapping his pencil on his desk, and sniffing constantly (considered a vocal tic, even though it is not created using the vocal cords) is thought to be willfully disruptive, when these are classic symptoms of TS. But because the child is not shouting obscenities or exhibiting other vocal outbursts, TS is never considered as a possible reason for the child's behavior.

The diagnosis of TS involves many steps. First, a parent or caregiver must recognize the symptoms. He or she must then consult a knowledgeable physician, preferably a neurologist who has had experience treating patients with TS. This is where the diagnosis becomes difficult. A child who doesn't understand why he or she is making these strange movements and sounds is naturally embarrassed when they occur. The last thing a child will do when he or she is brought to the doctor is exhibit these symptoms. Since the current diagnostic criteria for TS states that the symptoms must be present for a period of more than one year, a child needs to be observed for an extended period of time; otherwise, TS can go undiagnosed and untreated for years.

Because I was an adult, my diagnosis was fairly simple. I informed the neurologist of the symptoms that I had and the age at which they had started. I explained and demonstrated my motor tics as well as my vocal tics. He sat and discussed my symptoms with me, performed some other tests, and concluded that I indeed had TS. The first neurologist I saw informed me that I didn't have TS, because she never saw me tic during the visit. When she asked why I was so adamant about receiving a diagnosis of TS, I informed her that I had done some research and discovered that TS is genetic, and I was concerned for my newborn son. She frowned at me, expressed her doubts, and left the room. She returned with a child psychiatry textbook and looked up TS. She informed me that it mentioned nothing of its being hereditary. (In her defense, the gene linked to TS had not yet been discovered; but I felt that she should have been well-informed about current TS research as I was told that she treated patients with TS.) Also, she was obviously unaware of the ability of those of us with TS to suppress our tics. Needless to say, I did not return to her office.

Related Disorders

Attention deficit disorder (ADD), attention deficit hyperactivity disorder (ADHD), and obsessive-compulsive disorder (OCD) commonly occur alongside TS. Other conditions include, but are not limited to, learning disorders, depression, anxiety, aggression, asthma, and sleep disorders, such as sleep apnea and restless leg syndrome.

Due to these related disorders, TS is commonly thought of as a *spectrum disorder*. Please visit the Tourette Spectrum Disorder Association, Inc., at **www.tourettesyndrome.org** to learn more about TS as a spectrum disorder.

Medical Intervention and the Use of Drugs

TS is a disorder that is difficult to control by medical intervention. The most common method of treatment is medication.

Because I am not a doctor or pharmacist and have not taken medications for my TS, I will not get into a pharmacological discussion of each drug and its helpfulness and potential side effects. I will present some preliminary information to you so that you may conduct further research if you choose to learn more.

Because TS has until recently been thought of as a rare disorder, no medications are currently available to specifically treat its symptoms. Many of the drugs used fall into a host of categories, such as neuroleptics, anti-depressants and anti-obsessives, secondary serotonin reuptake inhibitors, sedatives, anti-anxieties, hypnotics, anti-convulsants, Alpha and Beta blockers, central nervous system stimulants, anti-manics, and neuro-toxins. This list is enough to confuse and frighten any of us; you can well imagine what it is like for parents who are considering medicating their child.

Speaking with the contributors to this book, and through my research, I have found that a drug used to control a patient's tics can have an adverse effect on her ADD. In other instances, controlling one's OCD can lead to an increase in Tourettic activity. It is a hit-and-miss philosophy. Combinations of drugs do sometimes help, but only after the dosage of each medication is tweaked until the desired effect is achieved.

Alternative and Natural Treatments of Tourette Syndrome

In recent years, there has been an increase in the use of alternative remedies for various ailments. TS is no exception. Limited studies indicate that dietary changes, allergy treatments, homeopathy, nutritional therapy, and other natural approaches have been helpful in controlling some Tourettic behavior. Please visit **www.latitudes.org** for more information on treating TS and other neurological disorders without drugs. *Latitudes* is the newsletter of the Association for Comprehensive NeuroTherapy, a non-profit organization dedicated to exploring advanced and complementary treatments for neurological conditions.

IN THE BEGINNING...

■ ■ ■

I chose the following five stories to introduce you, the reader, to Tourette syndrome. They encompass a wide range of symptoms, and therefore serve the purpose of showing the complexity and depth of our disorder.

THE WILL TO OVERCOME

Greg Blackburn

Twitch. Jerk. Twitch. Jerk.

Laughter surrounded me in a sea of desolation and loneliness. "Hey Jerky!" "How's it going, Twitch?" Hurtful comments, whispered behind me in the grocery store. Strange glares and curious stares at restaurants. Snickers from fellow teens at the church. All eventually stirred into the foul boil of the cauldron—one great stew of nastiness and pain. One great public chant, a mantra of mistrust and haughty irreverence for something called Tourette syndrome (TS).

Twitch. Jerk. Twitch. Jerk.

I heard the chant, the harsh truth of my being cast away from normality. They chanted jokes about a demon that claimed a part of my character. This truth that I speak of is potential pandemonium, waiting to pounce on victory, should I ever give into it. It is the pulsating convulsions of a neurological disorder that overwhelms its victims with grief and the agony and fear of others' harsh unwillingness to accept.

This neuron malfunction, Tourette syndrome, locks up its prisoners and doesn't set bail. Instead of the death penalty, it serves up a life sentence, without parole. This monster-jailer causes its inmates to jerk and spasm, physically, vocally, and

uncontrollably—day after day, year after year. It grabbed me
into itself and threw away the key.

The path of being different was paved for me as a child.
Vivid memories of being pushed aside from the crowd still
haunt me. Although these encounters, just sneak previews to
the real show, were hurtful, I always managed to keep my head
up high. TS, though, has an unusual way of eating at the emotions and causing mixed impressions. One minute you can be
on top of the world, and the next minute you're shooting out
tears for no reason.

Throughout my childhood and early teen years, the mystery of *Why Me?* would not leave my mind. In 1995 the question was finally answered. Thirteen long years I had pondered
on my twitchy situation, and at last I found the key. I'll never
forget the neurologist handing me that key, the key of a diagnosis. It was not the end, the final judgment, but it was a
beginning. Some people hold titles of prince or princess, but I
had received a special title: *Overcomer.*

I know this all sounds like an open and shut case, but the
judge hasn't heard the evidence yet. "Your Honor, I admit the
road to my diagnosis wasn't so easy. You see in the discovery
process of my misfortune, I had to undergo test after endless
test, and I was exposed to medicine on top of medicine. The
medications I was given had horrid side effects and caused
uncontrollable mood swings. I slowly grew apart from the *me* I
used to know, and became secluded from everything that mat-
tered the most. The medications drove me slowly insane."

It took some time to locate that flame of sanity that still
flickered inside my soul. I rekindled the banked ashes,
though—just in the nick of time. I stopped hanging by a
thread and took hold of the rope that could never be broken—
the rope that ties me to God.

When I grasped that unbreakable rope of faith, God

planted the seed of desire in my shallow furrow. The diagnosis gave me the first key to get away from my imprisonment, that imprisonment of viewing myself through the eyes of others. God gave me another key—not to just escape, but to flourish. This key is a four-letter word—*love*.

Through loving, not just others but also myself, I have grown to embrace—to appreciate and respect—the curiosities and even the fears of others. Through love I have come to respect myself for who I am. Love has taught me to keep my head held high and a big bright smile on my face. Instead of allowing a cloud to cast a murky shadow across my future, love has raised me above the cloud where the light shines all the time.

I have fought hard to accomplish my goals, even to excel beyond them. In a strange way, TS has helped me to strive for excellence. I want to show the world that a little jerk here or twitch there can't hinder one's ambitions. I am intelligent, and I have love in me. I ranked in the top ten percent of my senior class, attained the presidency of the National Spanish Honor Society, and was voted an Outstanding Senior. I am currently attending college and studying music and law.

Through the highs of these triumphs, there are still some valleys. But now, I see them for what they are and climb up and out. I will make it. With every stride, I keep my eyes focused on the tape stretched taut at the end of the course; and God keeps my heart focused on the process of every movement.

I have joined the game—and I'll see you at the finish line.

■ ■ ■

If you would like to contact Greg, you can send him e-mail at **kappasig-twitch@yahoo.com**.

THE COLLEGE EXERCISE

Allison Faith Zalaman

When I was nearing completion of my college studies, I was given as assignment to write a pathology report. I was told that I could write about anything I wanted. I chose to write an essay on Tourette syndrome (TS), and also decided to include a classroom activity that would open the students' eyes to the frustrations of TS.

I wrote down each motor and vocal tic that I could think of on a separate index card and handed one to each student in the room. I asked each student to perform the tic that was written on the card he or she was holding. While they were ticcing, I asked them to stop. I explained to each student that there is a difference between you and me. I asked you to stop and you did. But as someone with TS, I cannot stop. Trying to stop only makes my tics worse.

This exercise opened everyone's eyes. They said it was the most powerful thing they had ever experienced. My professor loved it and said she wished she had taped the exercise. After this project, everyone treated me differently. I only wish I had done this in the first week of school instead of during the last week.

I began ticcing at about four years old and was diagnosed at ten. I was too young to realize what the diagnosis meant, so I just dealt with it the best that I could. Since no one in my family has been diagnosed with TS it came as a shock to my family.

My tics were much more severe when I was younger. When I started taking medications for my symptoms, I began having seizures. I went to see a doctor but was not diagnosed with epilepsy. I am not sure if the seizures were directly related to the meds, but it seems that way because I stopped having them when I stopped taking the meds.

I used to blink my eyes, snap my fingers, and grind my teeth. I would roll in the corner between the wall and the bed and make barking and screaming noises in my sleep. I would also wake up in the middle of the night hitting myself. I would draw on paper to keep my hand moving, and was later diagnosed with panic-anxiety disorder. My tics waned when I was in my teens, but got much worse during my freshman and sophomore years of high school. Now all I experience in the way of tics is a shaking of my head, arms, and legs. I also get headaches and neck aches, so this tends to be bothersome. I currently do not have any vocal tics. I do, however, have a learning disability. I do not tic when I am working. I am a Licensed Massage Therapist and my work is my medicine. It soothes me and removes the urge to tic.

The worst part of my TS is explaining to others what it is because everyone thinks the disorder is always severe. I have been asked if I would get rid of my TS and I have to answer that I would not. When I was younger I hated my disorder because I had no friends. The other children's parents didn't let their children hang out with me. But now that I am older and wiser, I am proud to have TS. It makes me who I am. If I had three wishes, not one of them would include getting rid of it.

I do wish that people would be more understanding and ask

questions before making stupid comments. They should educate themselves; maybe live their lives in our shoes before they criticize us. Growing up I was always made fun of; knowing I had TS just gave others an excuse to be mean. I believed that folks who made fun of others were not comfortable with themselves, so they had to bring others down to make themselves feel better. With this in mind, I tried not to let it bother me.

I have two great parents—a mom who picked me up every time I got sick at school—and a dad who took off from work to come to the school and help me with problems. My dad always put me before his work. I would cry to my dad and he would reassure me. He would tell me I wasn't disabled and that I could do anything that I wanted to do. He was a wonderful man and would treat me as if nothing was wrong with me. My mom hated that I had it and felt bad. She also tried to do all she could to help. She comforted me when I cried at night. I had a wonderful support system.

My sister used to cry because she was upset about my symptoms. She felt bad that I had it and she didn't. Once when I had a seizure at school, my sister, who is three years older than me, found me on the floor, got really scared, and helped me. She was always supportive and helpful.

I remember I used to go to my grandmother's house in Florida during the summer months; I used to go to camp there and grandmother took great care of me. When I would wake screaming and hitting myself in the middle of night, she would hold me until it passed. She was wonderful to me.

I want to thank my mom, dad, sister, and grandmother for all the support they have given me throughout the years. I love you all very much.

TOURETTE SYNDROME AND OBSESSIONS

Robert Cook

I started reading at age eighteen months. My father had a compulsion to read aloud street signs while driving, and it resulted in my ability to read them very early on. From the time I was two until I turned four, my grandfather used to take me to a local donut shop in Georgia and make bets with the workers that I could read the menu. He never lost. My mother is a special education teacher, who ironically, now works with several children with Tourette syndrome (TS). She has helped diagnose at least one child with the disorder because of her experience with me and my father.

I was in an advanced program in second grade, and spent only a week in third grade before being skipped to the fourth grade due to my academic abilities the year before. I graduated high school at age sixteen, the youngest of a class of 306, and ranked in the top five percent of the class. In addition, I earned my B.A. at age twenty-one and my M.A. in History at age twenty-four.

I remember blinking my eyes and sniffing around age six, although my mom says that the first thing she really noticed was an arm-jerking tic when I was in third grade. I was diagnosed at age nineteen, during spring break from college. I came across an article in the sports pages about baseball player Jim Eisenreich, who has been very public about his struggles with TS. While reading the article, there was this feeling of total recognition as to what I had, and knowing that I was not alone with this disorder. I spoke to my mom about the article, and she mentioned that one of her students had TS, and his parents, both teachers, were active in the TS community. The student's parents recommended a doctor, and we went to him for a diagnosis. He spoke to both of us for a couple of hours, and diagnosed me with TS and obsessive-compulsive disorder (OCD). Several years later, I wrote to Jim Eisenreich, thanking him for helping me, in a way, to find a diagnosis for all these strange actions and feelings. In return, he sent me his autograph. I felt very relieved to be able to put a name to all the things I was experiencing and feeling over the years.

My motor tics include eye blinking, facial grimacing, head jerking, abdominal contractions, and shoulder shrugging. My head tics and a sniffing tic usually come out only when I am feeling very stressed. Other motor tics include licking my lips, constantly smelling things, especially my food, or an item that I am encountering for the first time. I have some touching tics, mostly the need to drum on my legs or tap my feet when listening to music, especially with a heavy beat. Recently, I've had a "jumping" tic—the desire to jump up and down over and over to relieve excess energy. I used to slap or hit myself on occasion when frustrated, first in the legs, later in the face. As a small child, according to my mom, I used to jump in the air and land on my knees. It might explain why I have slight knee problems now, even though I don't remember doing this.

My vocal tics include sniffing and throat clearing (this one fortunately went away late in my teens; it was a very annoying and often painful tic). I also have a swallowing tic from time to time that usually accompanies the sniffing tic. The tics tend to move from one body area to another every few months. This has become less frequent as I've gotten older; that is, the tics have stayed in place longer.

I have symptoms of echolalia—I repeat the last word a friend says or mimic an actor on television. I've gotten to be a pretty good mimic and vocal impersonator as a result of this. My classmates used to crack up constantly over my Howard Cosell and Robin Leach impressions; one of the positive facets of TS! I also exhibit palilalia and palipraxia. I often spend hours flipping an object around in my hand while watching television, bouncing my feet up and down, or squeezing a stress ball. I often repeat things I've just said, talk to myself constantly (which really disturbs my roommate), and make up nonsensical songs to sing for my amusement. My dad does this also. I can remember him singing gibberish phrases to my mom in the car as a kid—it drove her nuts! I also have a habit of making fun of television commercials and movies, making up fake dialogue over the real lines, or becoming indignant if something happens which could not occur in real life. Plot holes and stretches annoy me. I think I watched too much *Mystery Science Theater* and *Saturday Night Live* as a teenager.

I have a number of compulsive behaviors related to TS, including dislikes of certain clothing (especially turtleneck sweaters, anything scratchy, and blue jeans), and textures (anything soapy or greasy makes my skin crawl). I often wear the same articles of clothing until they are worn out, and frequently would wear the same items regardless of season (for example, shorts in wintertime). I even up when taking steps, having to take another step if it didn't feel right. I count objects compulsively, especially my cigarettes, pages in my notebook, and the number of lines on a page. I tend to collect and hoard objects, not throwing anything away as it might have some important future use I have yet to foresee.

I have collected coins, stamps, baseball cards, CDs, books, sports memorabilia, letters, and unusual art objects. I had obsessions with certain colors, to the point of demanding that all my food for a time be colored green. My mom would put food coloring into it to do that. I think it had something to do with the Dr. Seuss book, *Green Eggs and Ham*. I have to use the same type of ink pen (Sanford Uniball Gel pens recently, although this has changed), and get mad if I can't find them. I have "my" spot on the couch, certain cups that no one else can use. I get upset if coffee filters are left in my coffee maker. I always sleep in the center of my bed, having to use two pillows. Since I got a cat four years ago, I find myself checking on him constantly even though I know he's okay and exactly where he is.

When I get interested in a topic, I often become obsessed about it, spending hours reading everything I can about it, talking nonstop about it, writing about it, and feeling it. It's helped me get into subjects as a writer, and was a great help in graduate school, where immersion in a topic is not only common but necessary to survive. My biggest obsessions have stuck with me for years—sports (especially baseball and football), serial killers (to the point that my parents seriously worried about me as a teenager), politics, current events, music, movies, celebrities, artists, and actors. One of my friends described me as a knowledge freak—said I was obsessed with learning in general. I think it is an excellent description of me—I love to read, research, and discuss my obsessions, and it's made me a better writer. I've found that the obsessive aspect of TS and OCD has been a definite help in my choice of careers.

My OCD has actually gotten a little worse as I've aged. It mostly manifests itself in constant list-making and list-checking, as well as related anxiety. I am also slightly claustrophobic, especially in traffic (living in Dallas, this is not always easy).

Like my tics, some compulsions change—one obsession switches to another. I've found that almost all of them come back eventually, but some of my more severe tics and uncomfortable compulsions (especially self-destructive impulses) have gone away. I still have this one disturbing obsession. Sometimes I imagine, while I'm talking to someone, sticking a knife in them, usually in the eye. It's very unsettling. I'm not a violent person, and the people I am with when this occurs are almost always people with whom I am not upset in the least. It may just be that part of me that's obsessed with serial killers visualizing, but it's scary nonetheless. I don't talk about this very often as I don't think most people would handle it well, especially given my interest in killers. I have been accused more than once of being interested in these people because I secretly desire to be one, but this is not true. I think it's some dark fascination with dangerous people, extreme behavior, and obsession. There's a lot of obsessive-compulsive behavior involved in serial killing, and perhaps I'm just trying to find others like me in that obsessive mentality, although I (obviously) use it in more constructive ways.

There were times my dad told me to stop ticcing, which embarrassed me, but otherwise my family has been exceptionally tolerant, supportive, and helpful with my TS. The fact that my mom is a special education teacher probably helps here, along with the fact that we've had a lot of eccentric personalities on both sides of my family so they are used to tolerating peculiarity and strangeness.

My family rarely says anything or points out my tics, unless they are very severe. Then they express concern and want to know how I am doing. My parents have often found information on TS for me and I feel like they've done a great job of handling a child with TS. They rarely made me feel embarrassed, and never treated me like I was doing something wrong. My mom was always trying to find a diagnosis—she took me to doctor after doctor. One said I had allergies, another said it was a calcium deficiency. I think they were just as frustrated and concerned as I was about the unusual things that were going on.

My father has been diagnosed with TS in the last couple of years, although I don't see many visible symptoms outside of some facial tics. He's definitely very obsessive-compulsive, though—completely anal retentive. He, also, cannot throw anything away. As I get older, I find myself picking up a number of his compulsions, including mapping out routes while driving, compulsive list-making and checking, and some possibly Tourette-related anger problems. My mother also claims to be slightly obsessive-compulsive and has echopraxia. I have a younger brother with mild depression who currently takes Paxil *(Paroxetine)*.

My maternal grandmother was diagnosed with schizophrenia and depression in her thirties, and struggled with various forms of psychosis, schizophrenia, bipolar disorder, and dementia throughout her life. She spent the final two years of her life in a mental institution, which was very painful for the entire family. When she was not ill, she was a vibrant and intelligent woman. She worked as a pediatric nurse, earning two college degrees while in her fifties. In addition, my paternal great-uncle was believed to have undiagnosed TS, and one of his great-grandchildren has severe TS. My paternal great-grandmother Moore and her father were known as "peculiar" due to what the family called "Moore fits," which consisted of a number of Tourette-related and depressive-type symptoms. There are a number of other relatives on both sides who have had compulsive behavior problems, especially severe overeating and alcoholism.

My brothers both have a slight tic (one sniffs, the other squeaks) but they haven't been diagnosed with TS. We used to pick at one another's tics, but nothing mean-spirited—mostly just kids reacting to something unusual.

I am a writer and poet—I have written some poetry about my TS, but have not dealt with it very much in my work. Most of my friends are "artists" in some sense—writers, musicians, and painters, and I find from talking to them that most of them have had some psychological problems or learning disabilities at one time. Several of my friends were institutionalized for short periods before I met them. Although I did not know this prior to becoming friends with them, it doesn't bother me either way.

I think that my TS and OCD has been a positive influence in my writing career, and I've always known, on some level since I was seven or eight years old, that I've wanted to be a writer. My parents did a good job instilling in me a love of reading and education, and I guess it just translated naturally into a desire to write. I've been a voracious reader for as long as I can remember—my room is filled with boxes and shelves of books, and I've had a library card since I was seven.

I don't handle it well when too many things come at me at one time. I've worked a couple of jobs in telephone call centers, and the fast-paced, high-stress nature of the job is more than my nerves can take. My frustration and anger problems nearly got me in trouble a couple of times at work. I used to throw things when I got mad, and once I broke a thermometer at a restaurant where I was working. One of my concerns about my future with TS is having children.

■ ■ ■

If you would like to contact Robert, his e-mail address is **rc2671@yahoo.com**.

IT'S ALL ABOUT PERCEPTION

Rachel Arsenault

I first remember ticcing when I was about seven or eight years of age. It started with a head movement that looked as if I was swaying my hair out of my eyes. My mother still swears if she had cut my bangs, I'd never have developed Tourette syndrome (TS). That's a family joke; I used to tease my mom about it.

My tics got so bad at one point that I had to completely stop whatever I was doing, and shake my entire body as if I was doing the twist. That's one of my first memories of a severe tic, and I think it was around that time that I first went to see a neurologist. I was twelve years old.

The doctor didn't feel that he could confirm I had TS at that point because he noticed little or no vocal tics. He asked my parents to wait for a year, and if both motor and vocal tics progressed, then they should bring me back in. One evening, as my parents and I were chatting, they videotaped me. They had hidden the video camera in the corner of the room, so they were able to catch my tics in their true form. For some reason, whenever I went to see a doctor, my tics were never as bad as they were outside of his office, so this gave the doctor a chance to see how bad they actually were.

On August 23rd, 1993 I was diagnosed with TS. Believe it

or not, the only real emotion that I can remember feeling that day was relief. I can remember trying to explain my behavior to others in the months before my diagnosis. It was quite difficult, because I really didn't know what it was. I had suspicions that it was TS, but somehow didn't feel like I should use that as an explanation. Whenever I was approached by someone who asked about my tics, I'd say "Do you know what Tourette syndrome is? It's almost like that, except they're just tics." That worked fine for a while, but I was very relieved to be able to finally say, "The reason I make these movements is because I have Tourette's!" I've always felt that letting people know why I tic is easier than trying to hide it.

The motor tics I have experienced include shaking my body, twitching my head, blinking my eyes (the ever-so-popular), kicking my legs, punching (into the air, never hitting anything), shrugging my shoulders, snapping my wrist, wiggling my toes, and clenching my teeth. I have very few vocal tics, and never have I had the urge to utter words or obscenities; however, I do have the tendency to repeat things that have been said in conversation.

At one time, however, I did experience copropraxia. I had an urge to touch myself in an inappropriate manner. It was one of the harder things that I went through, as this tic occurred in public. It was just a quick gesture; however, it was something that I couldn't hold back. I hadn't thought about that tic for quite some time now, and looking back, I remember how painful it was to be mocked by other kids. I remember one specific incident, where as much as I tried to hide it, a boy in my class saw me do it, and brought it to the attention of the whole class. It was embarrassing, but I was lucky to have good friends for support.

Through the years I have had times where I've felt like I had to touch certain things or perform rituals. I remember for about a year, when I was about 15 or 16, before I went to bed, I had to perform this particular ritual. I don't know how I even came up with this, but before I turned off my light to go to bed, I had to look at the light, then the television, then the bed, in that order, over and over again. I did this twenty times before I felt comfortable enough to turn off the light.

I have tried medications to control my tics. The first one was called Dixarit *(Clonodine)*. I think it was a blood pressure pill, and my doctor believed that it would be one of the milder ones that I could try. It didn't work at all. The next one we tried was Orap *(Pimozide)*. Orap came as a recommendation from my ninth-grade teacher, whose son has TS. He had been taking Orap for quite some time and had found it very effective. I took Orap from about the time I was 14 until just a few months ago. I hadn't experienced any major side effects (apart from being sleepy every once in a while) until last year. I started experiencing anxiety attacks, where I felt as if my heart was sinking into my chest. This happened mostly at work, and was so debilitating that I couldn't do my job. I had taken almost a month off from work. I decided to stop taking Orap, and the attacks ceased. I try my best to hide or change my tics at work. Because I answer the phones, I can sometimes use my hands to disguise tics that would normally come out as vocal tics.

My grandfather had TS symptoms; however, he was never diagnosed. There are symptoms of TS on both sides of my family and I have one cousin who has been diagnosed.

My family has always been supportive of me. They are there when I need someone to talk to, and I'm sure they always will be. At first, as I think has happened to many of us, I was told to stop ticcing, but that was just because they wanted what was best for me, and didn't realize what was happening; I suppose I would have reacted the same way. As time passed, I opened up with my feelings and we learned more and more together. (I wasn't too shy to tell them how I felt!) I can remember one time when I received a chocolate bar in the mail from my aunt who lives far away. It was a chocolate bar that was in support of the Tourette Syndrome Foundation of Canada, and written on it was, "Keep the faith Rachel, they're working on it!"

My family, much the same as friends, became accustomed to my tics very quickly. I've had many people say, "I don't even notice them anymore." I think, from their point of view, TS isn't something that I'm affected by, it's just a part of who I am.

I was very lucky as a child in that I had a good group of friends that supported me throughout my school years, and that helped a lot. I remember a few times where some people were less understanding than others. My TS seemed to bother one boy in my class more than anyone. I remember one time, (not wanting to exclude me from class activities) my art teacher asked me if I'd like to pose for other kids to draw a still picture of me. In order to do this, I had to sit up on a chair in front of the entire class (which didn't bother me too much). This particular student spoke up, not too long after I got myself settled on the chair and said something to the effect of, "I can't draw her, she's moving all over the place." His comment hurt my feelings, but like I said, there were only a few people in my school that were like that. I gave presentations about TS to all the classes in my school. I told my story, explaining what TS really is, so that when these kids encountered someone else with TS, they'd recognize it.

One of the hardest things to deal with regarding this disorder is that it makes you visibly different, and that's the thing I struggle with the most in my life. The only thing I've ever wanted was to be "normal." I guess it's just realizing what "normal" really is. When you're a kid who's visibly different you don't feel normal, you feel like you're the only one stuck with this thing. And it's true, people do find things that are out of the ordinary to be "weird." Throughout middle school I had a good backup of friends; however, when I entered high school, I found it very hard to make new friends and found myself drawing back from social activities. I still did some things, but only things I felt one hundred percent comfortable with.

I don't yet have my driver's license, and that's mostly a personal thing. I had waited a couple years after I was eligible to get my license before I got up the nerve to go into the DMV to take the written test. As I sat down to write the test, a large gentleman came up to me and asked, "What are you doing with your shoulder, that jerking motion?" He was rude and impatient, hardly giving me time to answer. I explained to him that I had TS and that it was a neurological disorder that causes movements and sounds called tics. He told me I wouldn't be able to write my exam that day because I needed to take a medical and have a doctor sign it saying that I was able to drive. It wasn't a pleasant experience to say the least. Since then I've had a medical, and my doctor has said it is fine for me to drive, but I have yet to work up the nerve to go back to the DMV. (Silly, isn't it?)

I don't like sitting in audiences, so I haven't attended concerts or performances a few times because I didn't want to sit with a group.

I've come to realize that what people think about me isn't the most important thing, it's really what I think of myself. And what I think of myself is going to reflect on how people react to me.

COMPASSION THROUGH UNDERSTANDING

Shawna Rae Fross

I first remember ticcing when I was in first grade. I was diagnosed with Tourette syndrome (TS) at age twelve. I was crushed to find out I have TS. I felt like the whole world knew and would make fun of me for it.

It was the middle of the week when I was diagnosed and there was no way I was returning to school the rest of that week. While I was gone, my teacher, whom I did not like from day one that year, announced to the class that "Shawna has been diagnosed with a disease, and won't be back the rest of the week." I am convinced that when a sixth-grader hears "disease" their mind fills with all kinds of scary images. Three girls I had been friends with all year came up to me the following Monday during lunch to tell me they couldn't be my friends anymore because they didn't want to get what I have. And I thought being told I have TS was horrible! Silly me. After that, I remember many of my sixth-grade peers laughing at me one day at lunch because I was having a bout of really visible facial tics. I was very embarrassed by their laughing. I thought they were all very rude and I hoped, secretly, they would all burn in Hell for their behavior. I hoped that someday, somewhere, they would be publicly humiliated like they humiliated me.

The motor tics I have include winking and blinking, forcing a smile with my teeth showing, popping my jaw (both sides to make it "even"), stretching my neck muscles, twitching my mouth, wrinkling and wiggling my nose like a bunny, touching other people (on the shoulders, head, or arm), tightening my stomach muscles, shrugging my shoulders (sometimes doing it until they pop), smelling things, twirling while walking, making my fingers cross over other fingers without any help from the other hand, biting my teeth together hard and fast, licking my lips, closing my eyes when I am talking with someone, and jerking my head.

My vocals include making the "hmp" sound (quick and often high-pitched, sometimes starting low on the scale and working my way up as high as my voice will go), throat clearing, and stuttering and hesitating when I speak (I get an answering machine and I'm in trouble). Luckily for me, I have not experienced copropraxia or coprolalia, as I work with children for a career. That could be devastating. I have echolalia more than echopraxia but have occasionally found myself mimicking others' movements. I seem to imitate my own and radio DJs' words and voices more than others. I have palipraxia, and it lies in nicely with my obsessive-compulsive disorder (OCD). I flip a light switch, set my alarm, and lock a door three times. I know I also have attention deficit disorder (ADD) and attention deficit hyperactivity disorder, but neither has been diagnosed.

While in college at Boise State University I saw two psychiatrists regarding diagnosis of any or all three of these. Neither doctor would even test me because "too many people (mostly children) are being misdiagnosed" and they wanted to see the trends reversed. I was accused by one of the two doctors of wanting the diagnosis and intending to fake it to get the diagnosis so I could get "preferential" treatment in college and to "get attention." All Touretters are faced with a situation like this at some point, in which they are ridiculed for being who they are and having the symptoms they have.

ADD likes to go to class with me. If I don't sit near the speaker, my mind wanders where it will and I end up playing with my pens or reading something when I should be paying attention.

I use organizer-type bags and purses because my mind would go bonkers if I had a "catch-all" system. I become fidgety and quite wiggly if my interest is not captivated. I am not one who can just sit on a couch and "do nothing." If I'm watching something on television, it had better be funny or action-packed or I cannot sit still. I start feeling electricity running through my body and I am off the couch and pacing the floor while still watching the show. But when *Will & Grace* is on, get out of my way! I'm heading to the couch, and I don't want anyone to talk until the show is over.

I write only with blue ink (black when absolutely necessary) and I hate pencils. My CDs are organized not only alphabetically but by musical category as well. (If the stores can do it, why can't I?) My jeans are neatly stacked in my entirely-too-organized closet, blue in one pile, and all other colors in a separate pile. My shirts and skirts are very neatly organized. I use only white plastic hangers. Even though they are clean, I must keep the darks separate from the whites. Every wrinkle must be ironed out. Books have to be neat and well taken care of. I have to make my bed every morning. I keep a dinner menu a week in advance (maybe this one is more ADD management). I check my alarm clock at least ten times within the last five minutes of going to bed. The numbers must be dialed "just right" when making a phone call. My seatbelt must be worn if the vehicle is moving, but only after it has been fastened three times. Lights are turned on three times. The radio is turned on three times. The oven timer is set three times to "be sure" it is set properly. When coming off a flight of stairs, my right foot has to be the one to hit the main landing. That "Stop/Alarm" button in the elevator is very tempting!

As for my family, there is a young man about my age on my maternal grandmother's side who has been diagnosed. No one in my immediate family has been diagnosed, though. My dad and two younger sisters have both displayed symptoms, and on the occasions I pointed them out, they all became defensive and denied having TS. I don't mind having the only diagnosis. It makes me even more unique.

My mom has never displayed any symptoms and she has always been the least supportive parent. My dad has been my rock through all that TS has brought my way. Some relatives are annoyed, that's for sure. They are the ones who more or less avoid *Shawna the Freakshow* at family gatherings. I get a lot of quizzical looks from my own family when I start ticcing. My mom's parents have always been the most tactful about asking me questions about TS. They don't stare at me with a "Gee, I wonder if that hurts" look when I tic, like other relatives do. Some relatives, though they have known me for twenty-four years, still ask, "Why do you do that with your face?" These are adults I'm talking about here.

My dad always stayed cool as a cucumber when I ticced. He rarely asked questions and he always made it clear to me that I was and am no less of a person just because I have this medical condition. My mother, on the other hand, loved going to the bathroom to get a handheld mirror for me to hold and look into when I ticced. Of course, when I looked the tics would disappear at first. Then when one would build and build so much I had to let it out. That was when I saw the "freak" she saw. I was uncomfortable going anywhere with my mother because I knew I embarrassed her. My father's comforting words and kind heart were often outweighed by his lack of compassion. What my mother did to me made me feel horrible, worthless, and unlovable. My dad remains the most supportive but my mom is more understanding now. She gets flustered easily when I can't "get it out" while speaking or when I start winking or shrugging and popping my shoulders. That makes my tics even worse! My sisters still look at me kind of funny when my tics are flying left and right, but they've come to realize that the tics aren't going anywhere anytime soon and they're not hurting anyone. I am very glad they are as accepting as they are of my TS.

There have been times when my TS has waxed and waned. It was at its worst during the pre-adolescent years. In high school it seemed to calm down a bit, but went bonkers again when I started college. Undoubtedly, that was from the stress of not knowing what to do with all that freedom, and from having a thirty-mile drive each way during rush-hour. Since 1995, my TS has been mild compared to the earlier years, with the exceptional "bad" days. When my body is going through my premenstrual cycle, my TS tends to flare up, especially the motor tics (mostly facial) and the ADD. I have *no* trouble retaining water, yet have difficulty retaining new information and recalling previously-stored information. And then there is the obvious "stress" which causes all kinds of TS flare-ups.

From the time I was diagnosed at age twelve, to age twenty, I was on quite a few different meds for TS. I don't remember the order in which I took them; some were re-prescribed after another failed to work. I have taken Klonipin *(Clonazepam),* Catapres *(Clonodine),* both the skin patch and oral tablet, and Haldol *(Haloperidol).* Most if not all medications I tried made me very fatigued. I had a very hard time concentrating in school because I could hardly stay awake. If I remember correctly, the Klonopin increased my tics and made me very restless. Looking back, I realize the side-effects of the meds were worse than the tics the meds were supposed to control. I decided to go med-free in December of 1996, as a kind of experiment to see if my symptoms would be any worse than they were when my body built up the tolerance to each of the meds. I was very happy after about a month to realize my symptoms were not any worse; in fact, some of my vocal tics lessened. Knowing I had "freed" myself from my personal prison of meds, I felt major relief and I am happy to say I have remained med-free since then.

I enjoy writing and I am quite funny, if I do say so myself. I hand-write letters to family and friends, as well as e-mail them. I keep a journal, too. Writing allows me to express my feelings and thoughts about TS without having judgment passed on me. The reader can say or think what they want. But I won't let negative feedback affect me. Also, writing lets me get my sillies out on paper, which will hopefully be read and laughed over one day.

I had been fortunate in the dating scene. Before I decided to "go for a guy" I spoke with him for a while to get a sense for whether he might be considerate and compassionate. Sometimes it took me a few dates or phone calls before disclosing that I had TS. Once it was out on the table, I encouraged the guy to ask questions when he had them. All of the guys I had chosen to date had been very forthcoming with their questions and concerns with TS, and I appreciated that. My TS had never been the cause of the breakdown in any relationships I have had. I am currently happily married, proof that my TS cannot stop me.

My TS has also never impaired my ability to drive, although sometimes I zone out and miss exits. I much prefer standard transmission vehicles because I'm concentrating on shifting with my hands and feet and I don't tic so much. The only thing I can think of that my TS has ever prevented me from doing is sleep. Some nights my tics are so bad that I toss and turn all night and don't get a wink of sleep.

Luckily, my TS hasn't gotten in the way of my employment. Sure, my tics follow me to work, like Mary's Little Lamb, but they have never kept me from doing what I need to do.

We know that no two cases of TS are identical, and some of us have more severe tics than others. No matter what our symptoms are, or their severity, we share a common bond. We are each unique, and we have our choice of how we approach living with TS. We can hide from it, we can be ashamed of it, we can blame ourselves or others for our condition, or we can be proud of who we are.

Once you accept your TS as "a part of you," your view of the world changes. People are no longer "against" you. You will find many more people who are accepting of TS than people who are critical of it. When you are open about TS and share your experiences with others, you become a teacher of the ignorant. You might help someone to become properly diagnosed because you told the lady at the library about your TS and she has a niece who twitches without knowing "why."

Yes, TS can be a burden, but it can also be a blessing because we can use it as a teaching tool. We know what it's like to be the "different one," to be singled out. We can teach compassion to others by setting an example.

As far back as I can remember, I have been snubbed in public and at private gatherings because of others' ignorance of TS. Since the tenth grade, when I accepted my own TS, I have taken the opportunity to tell these rude people about TS by giving them a brief overview of TS without becoming indignant and snotty. My hope is that whether or not they show interest, they hear me, and maybe they will go home and think about it.

■ ■ ■

If you would like to contact Shawna, her e-mail address is **hoosierfross@yahoo.com.**

FOR THE LOVE OF PARENTS

■ ■ ■

The support of loving and involved parents is the key to raising children. The stories in this section will astound you with the degree of patience, love, and compassion with which these incredible parents have been blessed.

SUPPORT IS THE KEY

Teri Bernhardt

For my husband and me, Kevin's diagnosis was gut-wrenching. Like someone had come into our home and stolen the future we wanted for our precious son. We tried very hard to be strong for his sake and act like it was no big deal; however, privately we were devastated. There was so little information available on Tourette syndrome (TS) and we were desperate to know what to expect. We talked to local people involved with TS and they told us their own personal horror stories of what to expect from our son as he got older. It was presented in such a negative way that it only made things worse. We couldn't imagine our sweet-hearted, gentle Kevin turning into some uncontrollable, rage-filled child. It was just too much to handle.

My husband and I disagreed as to whether we should tell anyone, but I felt very strongly that we should be open and honest about it because making it a secret might make Kevin feel ashamed or put more pressure on him to "control the uncontrollable." We were lucky to have a large support group of friends and family, and the school was willing to do whatever they could to help him. In fact, Kevin was in second grade when a substitute teacher noticed his ticcing and called it to our attention. She had prior experience with TS.

I was already very active in the community, so word spread quickly and Kevin was enveloped with love and support from everyone—including his peers. We explained TS to his teachers and classmates each year in Louisiana and during our first three years here in Texas. We feel like we have created hundreds of "Tourette's Ambassadors" by letting his peers and teachers know what TS is and that Kevin is still just a regular kid. He emphasizes this after each "talk" by demonstrating his remarkable karate talents—breaking a board with his hand, arm, or foot. Occasionally he'll dazzle his audience with a flying-side-kick to break the boards (he's a total ham!). Several times during his talks, others in the room have raised their hands and said that they, too, have TS! It's such an awesome feeling to watch a child who perhaps felt all alone with his disorder, suddenly feel good enough to "come out" and feel kinship and acceptance. It has been a rocky road at times, but being open about his disorder has provided us all with the much-needed support and has lessened the load for Kevin as well as for my husband and me.

I do remember one situation here in Texas shortly after we moved. He was brand new to the school, and we had just had our "Tourette talk" with one of his classes. A substitute teacher noticed Kevin ticcing and she fussed at him to stop. He politely explained that he had TS and couldn't stop it. She fussed at him again and said that he could if he wanted to and that he *would* stop in her classroom! Well, this class of normally well-behaved sixth graders stood up and defended Kevin, which caused a bit of an uproar. It ended with a dozen kids marching with Kevin to the guidance office where this awesome counselor applauded them for protecting Kevin and had a talk with his very humbled and apologetic substitute teacher! Kevin's reaction: "I was thrilled that my classmates stood up for me, but I really felt sorry for the substitute teacher because I knew she just didn't know any better." Pretty amazing reaction for such a young child. That is still how he handles things. He's grateful for the support he gets, but understanding of those who don't know or understand.

Kevin's tics are usually moderate, but there have been times when his tics were severe. His most common "tic repertoire" includes nose twitching, eye blinking and rolling, mouth puckering or moving his mouth from side to side, eyebrow raising, hair flicking, shoulder shrugging, hand flicking or flexing, stomach muscle rolling (great for the abs), leg jerking, and little squeaky noises or throat clearing. Past tics have included shoulder slamming into the ear (bruised shoulder/ear—had to get x-rays), knee slamming (kneecap dislocator—more x-rays), severe eye blinking (couldn't see, had to be walked to classes), snorting (nose bleeds that wouldn't stop and a sore throat), arm jerking (tough to write), leg jerking (tough to walk or sleep), throwing up, and one complex vocal tic we dubbed the "donkey tic." Kevin wound grunt, then snort, and then squeak loudly. He *hated* that one, but fortunately it didn't last long and hasn't revisited him in more than a year. Right now he has virtually no tics and is not taking any neuroleptics.

Kevin has the whole alphabet soup: attention deficit disorder (ADD), obsessive-compulsive disorder (OCD), panic-anxiety disorder (PAD), learning disabilities (LD), including dysgraphia, and frequent bouts of depression (at times suicidal). He has frequent waxing and waning. Summer is his most tic- and symptom-free time (less stress, less tics). Usually a couple of weeks into the school year seems to be his worst time.

Kevin has taken several medications since he was nine years old. Below is a list that includes the name of the medication, the symptom it was used to combat, the age at which Kevin originally began treatment, and the outcome.

Catapres *(Clonodine)* for tic relief at age 9. Worked for a short time but increased his OCD.

Prozac *(Fluoxetine)* for OCD and depression at age 10. Kevin took this for four years until it lost its effectiveness.

Risperdal *(Risperidone)* for his tics and anxiety at age 11. This worked for about two years until Kevin began to gain weight and the drug lost effectiveness.

Orap *(Pimozide)* also for his tics and anxiety at age 13. After two months on this medication, Kevin experienced school phobia and vomiting.

Adderall *(Amphetamine/Dextroamphetamine)* for ADD at age 12. Kevin took Adderall for four months and it worked very well.

Klonipin *(Clonazepam)* for anxiety at age 13. He stopped taking it after three months because it didn't help much.

Zyprexa *(Olanzapine)* for tics and anxiety also at age 13. Worked for four months until Kevin began gaining weight and the medication caused an increase in his OCD symptoms.

Paxil *(Paroxetine)* for depression and anxiety also at age 13. He took it for a year and it helped the anxiety but did not do much for the depression or OCD.

Xanax *(Alprazolam)* for panic attacks at age 14. We tried this once and it made the attacks worse.

Seroquel *(Quetiapine)* for tics also at age 14. It didn't work well and after four months Kevin began to "see things."

He is currently taking Paxil at night and Prozac each morning. This combination seems to be working for the time being.

The meds he has taken over the years have kind of "see-sawed" his disorders because the tic meds seem to cause his OCD to flair, and the anxiety meds make his depression worse. As a result, his symptoms are constantly changing. We never know, though, if it's just his natural cycles of waxing and waning that are occurring or his reactions to the meds.

Kevin's grandma has just been diagnosed with TS and OCD and we suspect ADD as well. She is 69 and has had eye tics all her life. My two sisters and I have varying degrees of ADD, OCD, and depression, but no tics. One of my daughters has depression and ADD. Both of my sisters have OCD and depression. It's very obviously an inherited disorder.

We have had nothing but compassionate responses from everyone. It's actually been a relief to know what is wrong with all of us, however it hit my Mom the worst. She blamed herself for passing on "bad genes." I think we've got her over that feeling for the most part since it's not something she chose to have either! She gets very upset when he's having a rough time, though, and loves him dearly since they share a common bond.

We have tried our best to ignore the mild tics and comfort him when things get tough. Even his big sisters will snuggle up with him when he's having a rough time. He's super affectionate (we all are). I know that there are times when noises, especially, become frustrating for everyone. However, the girls don't complain, but occasionally will leave the room or come to me and boo-hoo because we all feel so badly for him. Sorry if that sounds "Brady bunch-like," but it's true. They love their little brother (who is actually taller than both of them at this time).

Kevin is taking his first art class at high school this year. He tried band, but here in Texas band is right next to football in importance and it was just too much pressure. He has a beautiful singing voice and a wonderful imagination. Karate has been a wonderful stress-reliever, and has helped him with body control and self-confidence. He holds a second-degree black belt in TaeKwonDo, a first-degree black-belt in TangSoDo, and various other belts in Hopkido, Akido, and

Jujitsu. He has taught classes at the studio, judges and partici-
pates in tournaments, and has been on demonstration teams.
He also loves other sports such as basketball and wrestling.
He's a WCW/WWF wrestling fanatic and is currently taking
classes with a professional wrestler. Kevin's done several shows
with Top championship Wrestling as the Cajun Kid and loves
being in the ring rather than just watching!

Kevin is popular at school and has girls calling him constantly. They are all fully aware of his tics and disorders, but he
has this totally charming personality that will win over anyone.
He's equally comfortable with his peers, younger kids adore
him, and adults are amazed at his polite manners and easy-
going style. He will chat with anyone and never meets a
stranger. He's "gone out with" or "talked to" so many girls that
I've lost count. He remains friends with them all. Having two
older sisters, he's been coached on how to be a gentleman.
They have taught him to open doors for the girls, how and
when to send flowers, and all the subtle things like saying the
right things at the right time. For example, when a girl asks,
"Kevin do you think I'm fat?" His answer is an immediate
"No," without looking below their eyes! He is trying to teach
his friends all of these subtle but *very* important tricks to keep
from getting slapped or dumped. Kevin can't wait to drive. We
haven't crossed that bridge yet, but we will be there in 18
months.

Kevin is currently on a partial-homebound program at the
high school. He takes his four main courses at home with a
wonderful tutor who comes in twice a week for two hours. He
goes to Art and lunch at school. He would love to be able to
attend school full-time like his friends do, but it wears him out
and causes too much anxiety and stress if he has to sit in a
classroom for more than two hours at a time. He had some difficulties keeping up with his work due to frequent absences or

needed breaks to the nurse's office to rest and regroup. He had a particularly bad eighth-grade year, so we are gradually reintroducing him to the classroom with electives only. He's very bright, but it's tough for him to keep up when his mind is constantly being dragged off task by OCD or ADD, or he is mentally or physically exhausted from holding in tics (or letting them out). His panic attacks and depression make it tough for him to get out of bed. Not to mention his frequent bouts of school-phobia. This "open-homebound" program is working well, since he is able to socialize at lunch and can go to dances and participate in other extracurricular activities. He can't play sports due to school rules of grades and attendance.

We are concerned since he isn't able to focus for long periods at school. Jobs can be incredibly stressful and finding a job that is flexible will be a challenge. He's young, though, and we can always hope for remissions, new meds, and miracles!

■ ■ ■

Teri can be reached at **teribern@aol.com.**

STEFANIE'S STORY

When Stefanie was six years old, it was very clear something was going on. Looking through old videos I noticed that it actually started at around age four. She was diagnosed at age seven. Even with all the research I did after her Tourette syndrome (TS) diagnosis was made, I was devastated. Knowing that there was something wrong that I couldn't make better was a horrible feeling. Stefanie and I sat and cried for hours that night.

Her tics are usually simple and they change frequently. Right now her tics include eye blinking, hand shaking, and head shaking. There have been so many tics along the way. I think that one that was most bothersome for her was "the cough tic." If I had to pick one we all liked it was the "kissing tic." Even though she "had to do it," all those kisses sure were great.

Stefanie repeats words and phrases to the point where she gets annoyed and wants to stop. Usually she repeats words to a song and sometimes repeats things others say.

It is not diagnosed, but as her mother I would say there are some clear obsessive-compulsive (OCD) traits in her. The way

---

*An asterisk next to a contributor's name indicates that that contributor wishes to remain anonymous.

she showers for example. Also I see that when something isn't "just so," she will do it again. This was very clear in kindergarten and first grade. Everything had to be perfect.

As her parents, the decision to medicate our child was not an easy one. With TS you have to "pick your battles" and decide what issues need to be dealt with. Stefanie's father and I, along with her doctor, decided to medicate Stefanie upon her first visit due to the fact that her tics were greatly affecting her "normal" routine. She was seven when she started on Tenex *(Guanfacine)* in December of 1998. We tried Benadryl *(Diphenhydramine)* for sleeping and that was a very big mistake. All that did was make her very, very irritable in the mornings. We started Catapres *(Clonodine)* in March of 1999. This combination seemed to work well for her with minimal side effects.

Stefanie's grandfather has TS but he was not diagnosed until after Stefanie was diagnosed. Her father also has OCD. Some of her cousins didn't understand in the early days; now everyone seems to have just accepted it. Some do ask and want to know, others don't seem too interested.

I have tried to be very educated and supportive from the start. We have had times when we just broke down and cried but mostly we try to have a very positive outlook.

Stefanie knows that she can let her tics go wild if she needs to when she is at home. I try to make her more comfortable when she is having a really bad time and help her when she needs help. She knows that she doesn't need to hide anything.

Patti was generous enough to offer a diary of her daughter's symptoms and medication regimen. This diary is so valuable, as it shows what a parent can go through as medications and their side-effects influence a child's tics.

September 1997

TS first appeared around September of 1997. She began shaking her head as if to get the hair off her face. She continued to do this even when her hair was up or short. Then, a short while later, she began to "skip" while walking. She would take a few steps then skip. The head shaking continued. Then we noticed other twitches. For example, occasionally her arms would "shake" and the head shaking changed form, but is still there. We began to hear her making "noises" if she was alone in her room or if she was upset. These vocal tics consisted of grunting, groaning, squealing, and occasional barking. This occurs occasionally and when she is under high stress.

September 1998

Stefanie's second-grade teacher mentioned at a parent teacher night that Stefanie has trouble staying focused and using her time wisely. She also mentioned that some of the other kids were saying things about her "noises," which apparently are much worse in the classroom. Also, she complained that her tics were so bad that she was unable to sleep.

November 20, 1998

We took Stefanie to her pediatrician for a physical. We mentioned the problem and suggested that we felt it may be TS. She would not make a diagnosis but did send us to a neurologist. The appointment was made with him for December 15th, and the diagnosis was made that day. The treatment plan included dosages of Tenex in the morning and evening. She began getting good nights' sleep after only the second night on the medication. Stefanie responded well to the medication, but this lasted for only two weeks. At Christmastime her tics got much, much worse. Mostly on Christmas Eve and Christmas Day. Her verbal and motor tics seemed much worse during this time.

December 29, 1998

I called Stefanie's neurologist and at his request we increased the dosage of Tenex. This seems to be working more effectively. Her tics do not seem to be as bad. We most surely do see a dramatic difference with sugar and sweets. She has changed her eating habits and she seems to have lost some weight. She is not as hungry as she was previous to taking the medication.

January 11, 1999

After being on the medication for almost a month we have seen great improvement in her tics as well as her social acceptance and her self-esteem.

January 22, 1999

Currently, she seems to be more vocal and much, much worse at night. She has had no bad effects from taking the Tenex in its current dosage. Although she takes a shower every night to help her go to sleep, this doesn't always work. Several nights this week she had great difficulty sleeping. At her visit with her neurologist, we altered her medication schedule slightly. He also suggested that we add something for the nights she needs help sleeping. Benadryl was the choice that was made. This did seem to help.

February 3, 1999

Last night Stefanie said she just felt sad and cried. Nothing particular was wrong, she just felt sad. We called Stefanie's neurologist and pediatrician today. Per her pediatrician's request, we reduced the Benadryl dosage because Stefanie has had a lot of trouble getting up in the morning for school. Mornings most definitely seem to be her worst time. She is usually very nasty and very much unlike herself. She tends to be very stubborn, very closed minded, and just nasty. Also her new tics seem to be more facial and upper body. Also her arm seems to tic very much. Right now this seems to be a bad time for her. I understand that there are ups and downs, and this seems to be a very down time (bad verbal and motor tics). Spoke with her neurologist tonight and he also said to decrease the Benadryl and if the sad feeling continues, that we should discontinue the Benadryl on Monday and call him.

February 18, 1999

Stefanie has been taking Tenex in the mornings and afternoons for the past week. We also added Catapres at bedtime. Her tics do not seem as bad as they were but she seems to have more mood swings and seems to get angry more often. She seems much more stubborn than ever before. She has mentioned on several occasions feelings of bad dreams. She at times does still have a difficult time falling asleep. She seems to have a need to be close to someone; it doesn't matter who, but usually she wants me.

May 20, 1999

Tics are minimal. She has two that stand out: her eyes and her right hand and arm. The bedtime dosage of Catapres was decreased, but she was not sleeping on this dose. Her school-work is still good. Social skills are not that great but they are okay. Excitement and stress most surely affect everything, especially her sleep. Temper-wise, she is much better. I think she almost knows its coming on and almost knows how to defuse it. Things are much better: she is no longer complaining of dizziness and also has not complained of her legs hurting. Overall, I would say Stefanie is doing well.

May 25, 1999

I guess I spoke too soon. The cough tic is back, she was home sick from school today: nausea, vomiting, and dizziness. This is the only tic that seems to bother her. Her overall atti-tude has been good. Her schoolwork is going well; however, she does seem to lack slightly socially. Not sure why that is, maybe that she just tries too hard to be a friend.

July 18, 1999

Stefanie has been doing well over the past two months. However, about two weeks ago her tics seem to have come back with full force. Her motor tics are much worse than they have been. Her tics now include the shakes, pointing her fin-ger, and blinking her eyes. She also seems to be very vocal again; grunts and groans. I think the cough tic is back. She is again having trouble sleeping: she tics in her sleep. Her temper also seems to be coming back. I called the neurologist on Friday. He is on vacation and will be calling back on Monday or Tuesday. Socially she is doing the same that she had been. She is a very smart, very aware child. Her appetite also seems to have increased again. I just wish there were something we could do to take her suffering away. She is so aware of what is going on and at times so very uncomfortable about it. I just hope we can go back to where she was without heavy medications. Well here we are again, the tics are still bad, and the temper is also. Not to mention the self-esteem. I think she is nervous about school although it's a month away. Socially she is doing okay. The same as usual I would say.

August 30, 1999

Okay, we are back to square one. The tics are back and worse than they have been in a long time. She is still taking Tenex twice a day and Catapres at night. Her tics were very bad after being at Nana's for the weekend. School starts on Thursday and that could have something to do with it, but I think it's something else. I think there was too much stress at Nana's. But it doesn't matter how or why, all that matters is we are hearing things like "Mom, help me cut this," and noticing a lot of things coming out that were never there before. Her tics now are more whole body than upper body and also seem to be more complex. There are most surely more muscles involved but fortunately they don't seem to be interrupting her sleep patterns as of yet. Taking into consideration all that is going on right now with school starting and sleep changes we are not going to panic. We are going to give it some time and see how things go. She is doing very well in so many other aspects that we want to see if her tics wane again. If and when she starts to complain then we will call the doctor. We called the neurologist on Monday and we were advised to increase the Tenex dosage. Stefanie's tics became less severe and things seemed to calm down.

October 1999

Things calmed down, for a while anyway. She began to get angry quickly, was very short-fused, very cranky, and uncooperative, especially at home; however, it was not noticed at school. At the end of September something happened that was so scary. Her neurologist said it was an anxiety attack. She backed herself into a corner, would not let anyone get near her, cried hysterically, could not breathe, and would not stop crying long enough to allow herself to breathe. I finally got her to calm down and breathe into a paper bag. That night when she went to sleep she was sweating so badly. On Thursday when she got up, she just didn't seem like herself. I have spoken to her teacher frequently and we talked tonight. She said last week Stefanie seemed to "not be there," but she is doing well socially, which is *great* news. Our plan for now is to decrease all of her meds and see how she does on her own. She goes back to the doctor on Tuesday. Hopefully we will get all this fixed.

November 1, 1999

Things seem to be going well. The medication decrease went well. She is doing well socially. She is "slipping" a bit in school, not sure why. She is just not the A student she has always been. She seems almost "lazy" about doing her schoolwork. She has not had a rage fit is about three weeks. There also have not been any more anxiety attacks. Her tics are minimal; not bothersome at all. There are some arm and facial tics, but nothing too bad and nothing that is interfering with her daily routine. She seems to be doing very well.

November 24, 1999

Where to start on this one? Tics are moderate to severe. Started today with a vocal tic that was just "cheep" over and over about every ten seconds or so. Doing well in school. Socially she is doing better in class. Her mood is changing at times and it's very unstable, though at other times it is okay. I have not spoken to her teacher lately but I know if there were any problems she would call. I called the neurologist on Tuesday and was advised to change the medication to Orap *(Pimozide)*. After reading up on Orap, we decided that the side-effects were too great and decided against it. Will see how things go after the holidays.

January 11, 2000

Tics are still moderate to severe. Her tics seem to be the worst they have been in a while. There is a vocal tic, the raspberry, which she hasn't done in a very long time. Her motor tics also seem to be much more involved than they had been; they seem more complex. Her sleeping is good. Stefanie is very much a morning person but she does well going to bed at night. She is faring well in school, both socially and academically. She will bring home another report card this week. Stefanie has had some major disappointments recently and has handled them well. She has not had any major rage fits, though she has had some minor ones. Overall I have discussed increasing her meds, but she doesn't want to.

January 19, 2000

Stefanie's tics are still very bad. She asked me the other day if we can increase her Tenex. I called the doctor and he said we could, but very slowly. We will increase starting today. I am trying to do things to get her more socially involved after school. She is having a tough time with her sister, who always plays with a friend, but not with Stefanie. Her anger hasn't been as bad since the med decrease. Besides her tics being so bad right now, she is generally doing well. Just to note, there have been two episodes that struck me as rather strange. One time about two weeks ago she complained of "pins and needles" in her head. Small area just above her left ear. This concerned me. I took her blood pressure and it was about the same as it usually is. This past Friday night she complained of a headache and dizziness. Also pains in her elbows and knees. This all lasted only for a short while. I again took her blood pressure and it seemed low but her tics were so bad that I had trouble getting it. She goes for a checkup today with her pediatrician to touch base, and I will bring her up to date on what has been happening with Stefanie.

February 9, 2000

There is so much going on. She said about a week or so ago that she doesn't feel the Tenex is helping and wants to stop taking it. I think its time for a change. She is very defiant with her father and me. She doesn't listen the way she always did. She "cries" at times for no reason. She has never said she is "sad or angry;" she just seems so all the time. She seems very distant. She is doing very well in school. She is also very short-tempered. Her tics are still much worse than they have been. She, however, does not have a problem with them. There is a whole circle of motor and vocal tics going on. Just noises currently, lots of repeating songs, words, and phrases. Stefanie also tends to be very loud and sometimes does not realize it. Another problem that we are having right now is she seems to never stop looking for something to eat. Currently, I think changing her meds will help and with a break coming up from school in two weeks, now is as good a time as any.

February 29, 2000

Well things are…things. Her tics are still bad, as is her attitude. She is still very unreasonable at times and very emotional; however, her tics do not seem bothersome to her. There are currently a lot of tics. Her arms are more involved than before. Some vocal tics are back again, just noises; the constant repetition is still there. Her facial tics do not seem as severe as they were. Her moodiness now is the biggest problem. She is still doing well in school, although some days getting her out the door is a chore in itself. There haven't been any more anxiety attacks and the rage fits have been mild. Overall, I guess she is doing okay. She is very anxious to play outside. I just wish she had some friends to play with. I will be calling Stefanie's neurologist today with an update.

March 8, 2000

So much is going on. Her tics are very, very bad, as is her attitude. She is also feeling sad again. Stefanie always looks like she is going to cry. Still doing well in school but starting to feel very alone and very "outcast." She has complained of her wrists hurting because of a new wrist-throwing tic. Her verbal tics are much worse than I ever recall; more frequent and more noticeable. I am also concerned that Stefanie is not sleeping properly. She is waking up at three or five in the morning and is unable to get back to sleep. This is, I think, part of the reason that she is irritable during the daytime. She does not seem to want to do the things that she normally enjoys. Sadly, she always wants someone to play with and there isn't anyone around. I am also having a very hard time coping with all of this right now as her sadness is very difficult for me. I called the neurologist on Monday. I have to do something and if it requires changing her meds, than that is what we need to do. We have increased the Catapres dosage at bedtime.

March 27, 2000

Tics are much better; different but better. Our biggest

problem now is her temper and her attitude. Stefanie does not listen. She does what she wants to do when she wants to do it. This is difficult for us and we do not let her get away with it. She is very stubborn and very disobedient. She is doing well in school as far as I know, but at home she is very defiant and very bad. Everyone that Stefanie sees on a regular basis has noticed the changes. Her medications are still the same, although today we switched to Clonodine, the generic of Catapres. That should not be a problem, so I am told. I called the neurologist today just to touch base with him and see where we are going from here. We need to have some idea what else we can do. We are willing to change her meds or do whatever it takes. We just want some answers and some help.

April 12, 2000

Tics are much better...usually. Temper is somewhat better. Biggest problem now is I think just kid stuff. Lying is a *big* problem now. Everything is "I didn't do it" even if she clearly did. Still doing very well in school. Socially she is doing the same. She wants to be involved; she just hasn't found a place to fit in yet. I am having a very difficult time with Stefanie right now as she refuses to listen to me. She has always been very open with me and this really bothers me. Not sure how to address it. Her dose of meds seems to working. She is doing well at night on the meds. Overall, she is doing well. There are just some things that I think we need to work on.

May 22, 2000

Overall, her tics are okay. In general, she is doing much better. Still a few things we need to improve on. Stefanie is very emotional and very nervous; otherwise, I would have to say she is doing well.

July 18, 2000

Current medications include Tenex twice a day and Clonidine at bedtime. Since school let out in June Stefanie's tics have been back with a vengeance. The lack of "routine" seemed to be a very hard change for her to make. The first few days were very hard. She was very moody, very cranky, and just outright very difficult. Her tics seemed to be more involved, more complicated. The medication increase has seemed to help her mood but not really too much else. I have also noticed that it takes her longer to calm down at night then it usually does. She has not been sleeping very well. She usually wakes up very early and has a difficult time getting back to sleep. Stefanie has a very wide range of tics now, some motor and some vocal. Socially she is doing okay. She tends to be very difficult, usually with her sister. She is listening to her dad and me at times, but we usually have to force the issue. Her tics seem to be almost non-stop. Mostly when she is playing her video games, is on the computer, or playing the piano. I have also noticed that she does not seem to have the control over them that she did before. We are noticing a lot more "tic-related spills." These make her very upset, although we don't get upset. I am hoping to get her calmed down a little before school starts again. She does not want to change her meds, nor do we want to increase the Tenex, but I think a change may not be such a bad idea. She goes back to the neurologist on the 24th. We will see where we are then.

September 19, 2000

Okay, time to bring things up to date. Stefanie has been doing well. Tics are minimal, temper had been better. She is doing well in school. Her current dose of meds include Tenex twice a day, Orap in the morning and evening, and Clonidine at bedtime. I have called the neurologist to see about decreasing some meds and making some changes as she had been doing well. Today was very bad. Today was the first day that she gave me a hard time to make the bus. She had a meltdown and I had to take her to school. I am not really sure what set her off but it was a clear setback. She finally did go to school, but it was not easy to get her there.

■ ■ ■

If you would like to contact Patti, her e-mail address is **hpynfreeny@aol.com.**

MY SON SEAN

Deborah Lynch

Sean started ticcing at age three. He was diagnosed at age five with obsessive-compulsive disorder (OCD), attention deficit hyperactivity disorder (ADHD), and at age six with Tourette syndrome (TS). His behavior was out of control and he didn't understand the diagnosis at all. I, on the other hand, was relieved to have an explanation for his behavior.

His TS is moderate to severe. It was mild when he was younger but as soon as he turned thirteen or so his tics got much worse. When he was sixteen, his TS was severe: full body tics, verbal, and motor—they literally exhausted him.

Sean has lots of variations of tics, they change every three months or so. When he was younger his tics included sniffing, blinking, nodding, making animal noises, clicking his tongue, kissing, twirling, poking, raising his cheeks, and smelling things, especially money. As a teenager they got more complex and more severe. He would hit his chin to his shoulder, bite his tongue, punch his leg, vomit, gasp, hold his breath until he almost passed out, inhale really fast, shriek, curse, spit, nod his head, spit into the dog's water bowl, and stomp his foot three times in a row. (Sean often does things in threes.) Sean has also exhibited coprolalia and echolalia.

Sean's tics wax and wane all the time, making it hard when trying a new medicine because we would think a drug was working only to realize his tics were waning. The tics get worse at holiday time and on birthdays. They are suppressed in new situations, such as when a new school year begins or when sleeping at a friend's house, but once he feels comfortable they come out in full force. They are bad when he is bored and restless, and seem to almost disappear when he is watching a good movie or playing a video game—something he can totally absorb himself in. Sean does not tic when he is asleep.

His symptoms change all the time. If the tics are mild, then the OCD is flaring. If the OCD is mild, then the tics get worse. The ADHD is always bad and has been his whole life. The rage was gone for about a year-and-a-half, but is slowly coming back. Some tics last a long, long time—the spitting tic lasted for over a year—but most change every three months or so. He does have the ability to modify a socially unacceptable tic—like giving the middle finger, or voicing racial slurs. Sometimes he changes them right in the middle of ticcing. Other times he trains himself to do something else—like when he is physically hurting himself while ticcing.

Since Sean was five years old, we tried various combinations of medications in an effort to get his behavior under control. Below is a list that includes the ages at which we started treatment, the name of the medication, the outcome, and any side-effects.

Age 5: Cylert *(Pemoline)* and Ritalin *(Methylphenidate)*; improved his ADHD but increased his tics.

Age 6: Mellaril *(Thioridazine)*; improved his tics but made his ADHD worse. Sean got paranoid and had nightmares. Benadryl *(Diphenhydramine)*; had no effect on his symptoms.

Age 7: Catapres *(Clonodine)*; improved his tics but made his ADHD worse. Sean was sleepy all of the time.

Age 8: Prozac *(Fluoxetine);* improved his tics but made his ADHD worse. Sean got depressed and suicidal.

Age 9: Dilantin *(Phenytoin);* had no effect on his symptoms.

Age 9: Haldol *(Haloperidol);* improved his tics but made his ADHD worse. Sean became paranoid, suffered insomnia, and experienced severe mental impairment.

Age 10: Klonipin *(Clonazepam);* improved his tics but made his ADHD worse. Sean became paranoid, confused, and agitated.

Age 10: Valium *(Diazepam);* had no effect on his symptoms. Sean became drowsy, confused, depressed, and experienced constant headaches.

Age 10: Ritalin slow release; his tics got much worse.

Age 11: Norpramin *(Desipramine);* improved his tics and ADHD. Sean experienced heart palpitations, agitation, insomnia, and headaches.

Age 12: Ritalin; improved his ADHD but increased his tics.

Age 12: Tofranil *(Imipramine);* improved his ADHD but increased his tics. Sean did so well that we kept him on it for two years; eventually the drug lost its effectiveness and made him very nervous and agitated.

Age 15: Tenex *(Guanfacine);* had no effect on his symptoms.

Age 15: Risperdal *(Risperidone);* improved his tics and his ADHD remained the same. Sean gained over one hundred pounds and we had to discontinue using it.

Age 16: Moban *(Molindone);* improved his tics a little and his ADHD remained the same. Sean experienced agitation.

Age 17: Prolixin *(Fluphenazine):* improved his tics a lot and his ADHD remained the same. Sean became restless.

Age 17: Prolixin and Pamelor *(Nortriptyline);* improved his tics but made his ADHD worse. Sean experienced agitation.

Age 17: Adderall *(Amphetamine/Dextroamphetamine)*, Prolixin, and Pamelor: his ADHD got much worse. Sean experienced extreme aggressiveness, anger, and frustration.

Age 17: Anafranil *(Clomipramine)* and Prolixin; had no effect on his symptoms. Sean suffered fainting spells.

Age 17: Zoloft *(Sertraline)*; had no effect on his symptoms. Sean experienced severe aggressiveness, rage attacks, and insomnia.

Age 18: Effexor *(Venlafaxine)*; had no effect on his symptoms. Sean suffered aggressiveness and rage.

Age 18: Celexa *(Citalopram)*; improved his OCD and had no effect on his tics and ADHD.

Age 18: Depakote *(Valproic Acid)* and Celexa; had no effect on his symptoms. Sean suffered restlessness, frustration, and aggressiveness.

Age 18: Lithobid *(Lithium)* and Celexa; improved his rage tremendously. Sean experienced diarrhea and hypothyroidism. (At this time we added Synthroid *[Levothyroxine]* to the meds list.)

Age 18: Zyprexa *(Olanzapine)*, Celexa, and Lithobid; improved his tics. Sean experienced another large weight gain.

Age 18: Ritalin slow release, Zyprexa, Celexa, and Lithobid. Sean's tics became explosive.

Age 18: Adderall *(Amphetamine/Dextroamphetamine)*, Celexa, Zyprexa, and Lithobid. Sean's tics again became explosive.

Age 19: Haldol *(Haloperidol)*, Lithobid, and Zyprexa. Sean experienced agitation.

Age 19: Seroquel *(Quetiapine)*, Lithobid, and Zyprexa. Sean experienced agitation.

Age 19: Nicotine skin patch, Zyprexa, and Lithobid; improved his tics and ADHD but wore off after a few months.

Age 19: Aricept *(Donepezil)*, Lithobid, and Zyprexa; had no effect on his symptoms.

Age 19: Paxil *(Paroxetine)*, Lithobid, and Zyprexa; the Paxil improved his OCD but wore off after a few months.

Age 19: Inversine *(Mecamylamine)*, Lithobid, Paxil, and Zyprexa; improved the rage, but it has since returned (I suppose the Lithobid is wearing off). The Lithobid dosage is as high as we can go, so we cannot increase it. The Inversine made the rage worse and did nothing for the tics and ADHD.

Age 20: Gabapentin *(Neurontin)*; Sean experienced agitation.

We have currently weaned Sean off of the Paxil, and he is now taking Lithobid, Zyprexa, and Synthroid.

In the beginning my family did not understand Sean at all. They thought he simply needed some discipline; however, as the years went by they have learned that it is not in his control and now they accept or ignore most of his tics and OCD behaviors. Our immediate family was always very supportive of Sean's TS—he was diagnosed early so he didn't have to go through years of having parents yell at him—we understand Sean. It is hard to live with the rages though; for those I have no patience.

Sean grew up in this neighborhood and his sister's friends used to wheel him in his stroller, play house with him, and teach him how to ride a bike. He was adored by everyone. When he was diagnosed, no one was allowed to play with him anymore; as a matter of fact, no one was allowed to play with my daughter anymore either. No matter what I said or tried to teach them about TS, it fell on deaf ears. One of my good friends at the time said to me, "I don't believe in Tourette syndrome. It's just an excuse to let your kid get away with misbehaving. Discipline is what your son needs." This was the saddest time of our lives. I found a good therapist for the kids and myself and time healed all wounds, but it did affect Sean badly. He was depressed for a very long time. We became "backyard folks" because it broke his heart to see the kids playing out front when he couldn't join them. But he did learn the value of a real friend and that was a valuable lesson in the long run.

Our daughter, Erin, was dealing with her own issues of OCD when she began having difficulties in school due to the stress that Sean's diagnosis was causing her at home. I had a meeting with all of Erin's teachers and explained why Erin was having such problems. One of the teachers remarked, "I think you should put your son in an institution if his Tourette's diagnosis is affecting your daughter."

Sean's TS gets in the way of him socializing with "normal kids." He gets teased and taunted just walking down the block. Sean is 21 and has never been out on a date. When he likes a girl and is near her his tics get so bad he has a hard time even talking. He gets depressed over this sometimes, but is usually okay with it. He attended a school in which half of the student population had TS. So, for the first time in his life he was accepted in school and was able to make friends. I truly believe that this school saved Sean's life.

Sean has only had four jobs in his life. At all four he had a problem with teasing, and when Sean is teased his tics get worse. His spitting tic was the worst as far as work was concerned. It was the one tic no one understood, accepted, or tolerated. He ended up calling in sick so much that he would get fired.

In July we signed up with Community Enterprises, an organization that teaches kids like Sean to write resumes, go on interviews, and get jobs. They have a shadow program where they are assigned to a worker and that worker walks them through the steps of applying for a job, going on the interview, and then once they get the job, the shadow is there to make sure they know what to do. Sean has always had a problem with remembering his job responsibilities. He was assigned to a pretty young girl who is studying to be a social worker. I think she was trying to get experience working with kids like Sean. Sean really liked her, which was a big plus because if Sean really likes someone he tries much harder. They went on interviews for months. She helped him type up a resume, taught him how to fill out job applications, taught him how to follow up on applications, did some transportation training with the public buses, and showed him how to dress appropriately for job interviews.

Since we split his classes in half last year, he only had to take a few classes in September, so he got out of school at eleven-thirty and was home an hour later. Then his shadow would work with him for a few hours a day. This did get off to a rocky start because Community Enterprises was short-staffed and there were weeks that he didn't get any services from them whatsoever. Just Sean's luck. By December he was frustrated, to say the least, and after raising holy hell with them, 2001 turned out better for him.

Community Enterprises found Sean a job at a Kaybee toy store in Westbury. Kaybee really liked him and said he was a good worker, which was praise that he had never heard before from an employer. He liked the people, the work was easy, and he was learning to use the transportation system here on Long Island. The school bus brought him to work and he took public buses home. He had to learn how to transfer buses, which sounds easy to most people but it was an ordeal for Sean. All the bus numbers were mind-boggling to him. Even with schedules in hand he got confused and we had to pick him up many times from someplace he should have never been, but he has learned a lot. Sean had to quit Kaybee because they couldn't offer him more than three hours of work a day. Sean needs to work full-time every day; all he does is sleep when he has nothing to do. We eventually had to leave Community Enterprises in January as they could no longer find Sean a job.

Another problem we had was with the educational system. New York State implemented Regents tests for all high school students. Although he graduated high school in June, he had to continue with summer school to pass the Global Study and U.S. History Regents competency tests. He failed the Global Study test twelve times. Even with untimed tests, testing in a separate location, and the use of a scribe, Sean was unable to even come close to passing. Very discouraging. I didn't want him to settle for an Individual Education Plan diploma; I wanted him to earn a regular diploma. After a most difficult summer, he finally passed the Global Study test. I think it is unfair to make special-ed students take the same tests as regular students just to get a High School Diploma. He passed the U. S. History Regents in January and Sean now has a regular High School Diploma. We are all very proud of him.

These tests are a pet peeve of mine. I did very poorly in high school. In fact, I think the only reason I graduated was so the school could get rid of me. I went back to college the same year Sean was born, and it took me nine years to get my AAS and six more years to get my BS. But I did it, and I did it well: I graduated with a 3.85 GPA. I never had to take these Regents tests; to me these tests are a waste of tax-payers' money and time. All the teachers do all year long is prepare the students for these tests, over and over, and the kids could be learning so much more if they didn't have to practice by rote for these tests. I cannot count all the letters I have written to Congressmen about this issue. I got nowhere.

Now that Sean has passed these tests, he moves on to Vocational and Educational Services for Individuals with

Disabilities (VESID). They have two programs. The first one is a shadow program similar to Community Enterprises, and the second one is vocational education where they will pay for him to go to a school and learn a vocation.

Sean wants to be a professional make-up artist, but I told him that is a field in which it is very difficult to get an education and find a job. I was able to talk him into learning how to program computers. This is something that is more realistic, and I told him he can put his dream on hold for the time being. At least he would learn something he could apply in real life, and VESID would pay for this schooling. I am also looking into scholarship grants to send him to Tom Savini's make-up school in Pennsylvania.

The Lithobid does little for Sean's rage. He gets angry and uptight over everything, making it hard to feel sorry for him as you might imagine. TS is not such an issue anymore, as his tics have calmed down and are minor compared to what puberty brought on. He has a few tics that are hardly noticeable; nothing so severe as to do him injury, and they have taken a back burner to his rage.

I often wonder—is the rage from the TS or is it a result of Sean's bipolar disorder? His doctor has no idea what to do next. We just increased the Lithobid because his last level was on the low side, but I don't see any improvement at this time. He is increasingly harder to live with, has no regard for other folks' property, or feelings for that matter, and after a rage he literally falls apart right in front of us. It is more depressing now because we always hoped maturity would help.

We took him off the Celexa, as I think it was aggravating his rage, and I want to try switching the Synthroid to the natural form of thyroid hormones that has TSH in it, as well as T3 and T4. It is not synthetic; it is derived from pig thyroid. From what I have read, kids like Sean do better on this new drug as far as mood is concerned. The Synthroid just might be inducing the rages and we will see the endocrinologist again.

The TS all by itself is not that bad—it is society's reaction to it that will break one's spirit. Being teased and taunted is like a knife in the back and can cause a person with TS such heartache and pain, and could very well lead to depression and suicidal thoughts. If society only knew the pain that teasing causes; if society did understand, maybe it would be more accepting of someone who is "different." It is so easy to say "stop it" to someone who is ticcing; it is a lot harder to ignore it and see the person behind the TS. My son complained to me once that no one knew him as Sean—they only knew him as "ticboy"—and that really bothered him. The schools don't understand either. I once told a teacher, "Why don't you try looking beyond the tics and try seeing the little boy underneath the Tourette's. You just might like him!" Her reply to me was, "If he would just stop doing those *things,* maybe I could." No one understands.

Sean recently got a job making carpets for automobiles. He works with two of his uncles and another employee who has TS. Sean has finally been accepted as one of the guys. This is truly a job made in heaven for him. He is much happier now. He has begun to mature and become responsible and is turning into quite a nice young man. It seems his rage decreased as soon as he was accepted at his new job.

■ ■ ■

You can send Debra e-mail at **dlynch32@aol.com.** *Please feel free to also visit Debbie's Web site at* **mysonsean.homestead.com.**

MY PRECIOUS GIFTS

Arthella Carpenter

Michael was about three when we first noticed what later turned out to be tics. At the time we just thought they were noises that children make. He was diagnosed with Tourette syndrome (TS) at age 9. He has also been diagnosed with attention deficit disorder, bipolar disorder, oppositional-defiant disorder, panic-anxiety disorder, and obsessive-compulsive disorder.

He just knows he is different. Many times he feels like an outsider. He doesn't understand why he has intrusive thoughts, and why he cannot retain information, for instance, school work. He gets really frustrated just trying to do his work. He has very slow, sloppy, and painful handwriting. I know that he hallucinates, but he will deny this to anyone because he is embarrassed for anyone to know.

Michael has a wide range of tics. He hits himself, jerks his head, shrugs his shoulder, taps pencils, and gets up and walks around in a circle. He spits, smells everything he drinks and sometimes eats, has to touch almost everything he sees, and runs into things because he does not watch where he is going. He also grunts, yells, sucks his lips, repeats himself continuously, cries, and says he can't catch on. He vocalizes his frustration in many different ways. His tics are bad and they are getting worse as he gets older.

Michael has no fear of danger. He will throw himself to the floor and hit his head on the wall or on concrete; he doesn't care. It is like his mind is saying do this and he cannot stop. He will cry loudly and pull his hair out by the handfuls. He sucks on his shirts a lot. He has problems remembering, and has a lot of panic and anxiety attacks. He also gets a lot of stress headaches and stomachaches.

He has a lot of problems remembering things such as putting on his deodorant and brushing his hair and teeth. Since he got braces, he has been better at brushing his teeth. His orthodontist told him no matter how hard he brushes the braces will not fall off. Michael took that as he has to brush really hard and he brushes his gums raw. I have to remind him daily to take care of his personal hygiene.

The school states that Michael does not qualify for the Individuals with Disabilities Education Act (IDEA), so they have him under a 504 due to his nut allergies; it is like they are ignoring his symptoms. As his parent, I cannot ignore the pain and suffering he is going through. He struggles so much. According to the school I am a trouble maker because I will not give up and I continue fighting to get my son the education he deserves. I work with him anywhere from two to six hours each night with his homework. I write notes to the teachers stating that he is not understanding the work and I get responses back like, "We went over this in class." The teachers don't care. They just want to pass him along and get rid of him. I want him to be self-sufficient in life.

Michael's tics still wax and wane a lot. The school says they don't see it happening there. I also want to add that I have brought up at several 504 meetings that Michael may ace his spelling test and in a day or two he forgets how to spell the words. The attitude I get from the school is as long as he does well on his test and can sign his name, then that is all he has to be able to do.

We have given Michael many medications to try to control his symptoms. He has been on Ritalin *(Methylphenidate)*, Catapres *(Clonodine)*, and Depakote *(Valproic Acid)*. The Depakote caused seizure-type symptoms. He has also taken Tofranil *(Imipramine)*. He is currently on Gabapentin *(Neurontin)*, Wellbutrin *(Bupropion)*, and Zyprexa *(Olanzapine)*. I don't think he has been on the correct medications for his disorders.

The hardest part is standing by and watching my son go through the teasing. Because of his learning difficulties and self-injurious behavior, he doubts himself and says he is dumb.

I wish that everyone who has to deal with children with TS or any other disorders would attend in-services regularly to educate themselves on how to better help the child. People without TS tend to think that when a child or adult is ticcing, they are crazy. Additionally, whenever a parent tries to remove his or her child from a store because the child is ticcing uncontrollably, others around seem to assume that the parent is abusive towards the child. I have even had people call the cops when Michael has had screaming episodes. Of course by the time the police arrive, Michael is usually calmed down. When the officers question him as to why he was screaming, Michael just gets embarrassed and usually responds that he doesn't know why and then proceeds to tell them to go away and leave him alone.

I also believe we need to help the child or adult with whatever problems they may have rather than look down on them. We need to be understanding and patient first and foremost, and not judge them for things they cannot control. Putting ourselves in the parent's shoes occasionally might even help us to perhaps understand what they are actually going through.

Everyone in our family understands that Michael has tics and we try not to bring attention to them because it makes him feel very uncomfortable. I am very protective of both my children and will do all within my power to not let anyone discriminate against or make fun of either of them. I know other kids at school still tease Michael, and even his brother Carl teases him when he gets angry at Michael. Whenever I can, I quickly put a stop to the fighting and bickering between them, but I know even this affects Michael as I often have to go to him and calm him down.

I love both of my children, and would never trade one moment of memories that I have had with them. Michael may have disorders, and at times I do become overwhelmed with all we have to deal with, but even with all the problems, I count my many blessings daily. God knew what he was doing when he gave my children to me and I know that He would not have given me more than I can handle (with His help). I will always be here for Michael at whatever age and for whatever he needs me. Michael's biological father left him when he was very young and he deals with a fear of loss on a daily basis. I constantly have to assure him that I will never leave him and whenever it is my time to leave this earth, I will still watch over him and walk by his side even from the other side.

TOURETTE SYNDROME IN THE FAMILY

■ ■ ■

The genetic component of Tourette syndrome is alive and well in many of the stories in this book, but nowhere is it more evident than in these three accounts.

A FAMILY AFFAIR

Vicki*

My diagnosis came about in an unusual way. When our nine-year old daughter started exhibiting symptoms, we took her to the neurologist. When I asked if she had Tourette syndrome (TS), the doctor said, "Why, sure she has Tourette's, and she inherited it from you. You've snorted three times in the last fifteen minutes." For the life of me, I couldn't recall one single snort! After our diagnoses (our daughter is a fraternal twin; her sister shows no symptoms), I became more educated about TS. I could look at each family member and point out every tic.

Armed with this new knowledge, I came to realize that my family has a definite history of TS and obsessive-compulsive disorder (OCD). My father, who was posthumously diagnosed with TS, had many tics that included finger drumming, foot shaking, leg bouncing, and rattling the change that was in his pockets. I believe that he had coprolalia, and though he never actually used profanity, he would say things in very poor taste at the wrong time and in the wrong place.

My paternal aunt has TS and OCD. My mother has never

---

* *An asterisk next to a contributor's name indicates that that contributor wishes to remain anonymous.*

been diagnosed with TS or OCD, but she shows definite symptoms of both.

My brother was diagnosed with TS when he was thirty-six years old. It was a nightmare living with him. When we were growing up he constantly moved, touched, twisted, and generally annoyed anyone in the same room. He also has attention deficit hyperactivity disorder (ADHD), and though smart as a whip, he is unable to sit and concentrate long enough to learn.

I taught my brother his ABCs on the swing set in our backyard, singing each letter with rhyming words for every forward swing. It was as if he had to be in motion to allow his brain a chance to absorb whatever the lesson was. I don't recall him ever taking medications except for asthma. He currently has a facial tic where he moves his eyeglasses up his face, dips his chin as he slides the frames back down his nose, and then starts moving them back up his face using only his facial muscles. Try that one!

As an adolescent, our daughter had vocal and muscle tics from her nose to her toes. Her tics are moderate now, either due to the medications she has been taking or just to the passing of time. But even on the highest medication dosage she still shrugs her shoulders and neck, flexes her hands, and blinks. Her OCD can interfere with normal family interactions. Hormonal swings tend to make her more volatile and less patient.

My oldest son (he is 19) has to touch or hug me, always telling me he loves me. Often, he does this ten or more times before he goes to bed at night. He also has to touch his sisters in some way, usually enticing some sort of frustrating response from them. Is this just sibling interaction or is it some form of TS? I would venture to say TS because of the family history.

I first remember ticcing at age 8, but was not diagnosed until I was 38. Still, I was surprised, horrified, unbelieving, and ashamed. My tics have included hair twisting, neck and shoulder shrugging, head twisting, sighing, and ho-humming, which I incorporate into singing or humming, so it is less noticeable.

I also have this uncontrollable urge to disclose details about certain experiences in my life. This can and has been especially embarrassing if my secret is of an intimate nature. I was horrified to hear myself describe some sexual experimentation between my husband and me. I blurted it out to a large group of acquaintances at work. It's not just an inability to keep a secret; it's a compulsion to blab those details best left unsaid. I don't have any difficulties keeping a secret such as a birthday gift or surprise for someone.

I feel intense anxiety in some social situations and I have a fear of heights. This fear is not due to the height itself, but an overpowering urge to jump. Consequently, I do not trust myself in high places.

I have not taken any medications for my TS. I have found that practicing relaxation and biofeedback works best for me. Long before I was diagnosed, I learned to use biofeedback to quiet and relax sore muscle groups I was using for a specific tic. I also learned how to shift my personal tic compulsion to another muscle group to give sore muscles a break. This is certainly not fool-proof and may not be for everyone, but I have had moderate success with biofeedback. It costs nothing and is easy to do.

We have also had our struggles with the school system. What teachers need to understand is that TS is a disorder with varying degrees. Most cases involve hidden symptoms or compulsions. Just because we can hold back a tic for a few minutes, we are still struggling with the compulsion to do that tic. Try to be more open to understanding that our role here is not voluntary. We can no more stop ticcing than you can stop breathing. Sooner or later it's going to happen. It's hard to say what an individual's needs are, but realize that with TS those needs change constantly. Just being flexible would be a great start. In a structured school situation it is very difficult to be flexible for one child and not the others, especially if it's a case where the tics are not as much a factor as the compulsions or the ADHD.

■ ■ ■

Vicki can be reached at **sugar4559@hotmail.com.**

GENERATIONS

Marlene Remley

I am a fourth-generation ticcer. My mother has Tourette syndrome (TS), as did my grandmother and great-grandmother. I also have a great-aunt that has TS.

I first started having mild tics at about four-and-a-half years old. My parents noticed them and took me to my pediatrician, who suggested that we visit the Movements Disorders Clinic at Oregon Health Science University. From there we went to the Genetics clinic, where I was diagnosed with TS and a learning disability. I was five years old.

My family has been fairly understanding of my tics. My parents don't really react to my tics now because they are so used to them. When I was little, however, they were overprotective of me and wouldn't let me do the things that my girlfriends were doing. My relatives pretty much ignore my tics, and treat me as if they don't exist. However, if they see my tics getting out of control, they will say something about them. Since I was five years old, I have been prescribed Haldol *(Haloperidol)*, Catapres *(Clonodine)*, Cogentin *(Benztropine)*, Valium *(Diazepam)*, and Klonipin *(Clonazepam)*.

My husband pays very close attention to my tics and when he sees that I am ticcing a lot, he makes sure that I get more rest and less stress. My husband is very supportive of me and all the things I aim for in life, more so than my parents ever were. I have two daughters, neither of whom have shown any symptoms.

I was made fun of all through grade school. Junior high school and high school were sheer agony. Kids were incredibly cruel to me, picked on me, harassed me, and tried to pick fights with me.

High school is where I learned I had to either fight or get the stuffing beat out of me by the other kids in school. I did not have a lot of friends, but the few I did have were really truly friends. They stuck by me no matter what. Even after graduation we stayed in touch.

The only thing TS has prevented me from accomplishing is getting a job. When employers see me they tend not to hire me. So I have no real job skills as of yet. However, I am currently in college full time working towards a degree as a Legal Assistant. I hope to be able to get a good job and make myself a better informed individual about the legal rights of the disabled.

A FAMILY HISTORY

Eileen Kelly*

Most of my immediate family is in denial about Tourette syndrome (TS). They think this is just something I am making up. They do not think any of them have it either. And of course they do not think their perfect children have it. As I sit at family gatherings, watching the eye blinking, listening to the grunts and throat-clearing, I chuckle to myself.

My parents are somewhat supportive. I think they are slowly starting to see that maybe they have some of these symptoms. They have always been very protective of me and my "problems," and they are fairly protective of my son, too. My mother will say, "Oh, your tics are really bad tonight," or mention that my son's tics are really bad today. She doesn't pass judgment on us. My dad doesn't notice much. However, when there are family gatherings, all hell breaks loose. There is usually some sort of disturbance—either between me and a sibling, or between my son and a family member—that can get pretty nasty and violent. Many times I have had to grab my two-hundred-and-twenty-pound son and wrestle him away from one of his cousins. Of course, he is blamed for anything

* An asterisk next to a contributor's name indicates that that contributor wishes to remain anonymous.

that happens, and sometimes the parent of that particular child and I get into it.

My husband has put up with a lot from me. I raged at him for fifteen years; luckily he has stuck by me. And when my youngest son came along, my husband took it from both of us, and it wasn't fun. Prior to meds, I had a huge blowup with my husband at least once a day. I was violent, abusive, nasty, inflexible, and I couldn't stand the least amount of change. I can only say that I am glad that I got help. We have spent a fortune on family counseling over the years.

Even as a child, my temper had a reputation of it's own and not many people dared to look at me the wrong way. I was always getting into fights and even though I was very small for my age, kids were scared of me.

I lost my temper on a regular basis. I was always blurting out things, and frequently said the wrong things to the wrong people. Fortunately, I was cute and got away with a lot. I was a tiny girl and when someone would accuse me of beating anyone up, I don't think people believed it. I got in trouble only once in school. I was always kissing boys though, and that was noted on several occasions.

I first remember ticcing when I was around eight years old. I used to scrunch up my nose and sniff. To this day, this is the one tic I try really hard to control. If I even think of this tic, I want to do it. My parents, particularly my mother, hated this tic. She used to tell me it made me ugly. I still bear the scars of that treatment. I am pretty well terrified of doing one tic for fear I won't be able to stop. They sent me to the doctor and he said I probably had allergies.

I was 35 years old when I was diagnosed with TS and obsessive-compulsive disorder (OCD). My eight-year-old son was having a lot of trouble and at the insistence of the school, we took him to a child psychiatrist. During the appointment, I jokingly mentioned that my Mom had said, "Maybe he's got Tourette syndrome." The doctor said, "Well, actually I think that is what he has, and I think you have it too." Well, I can tell you I was in shock. He did not want to make the diagnosis himself so he sent us to an expert on TS. It took six months to get an appointment, at which time he confirmed the diagnoses of TS and OCD for me, and TS, OCD, and attention deficit hyperactivity disorder (ADHD) for my son. Later, I was also diagnosed with sleep apnea and restless leg syndrome. After the shock wore off, I felt tremendous relief for both of us. I had always thought that I was either schizophrenic or manic-depressive, so it was a relief to me to find out what has been wrong with me my whole life. It all made perfect sense.

I think I have a fairly severe case in that it has adversely affected my life. My tics have been well hidden over the years, and most people just think I'm weird and that I have allergies. My rage, however, was a different matter. I was always fighting with people. I used to get into fights with people on the street and while standing in lines. I've had people strike me. I have hurt friends, family, loved ones—and my poor husband has put up with a lot.

I never really fit in very well. I always felt like an observer. I still feel isolated in crowds. Because of my fear of blurting out things, I used to clench my jaws so I wouldn't say anything embarrassing. This has caused me to have neck problems. Now that I'm on meds, I feel much better about myself and feel more comfortable. I have always had a great sense of humor, and that used to help me in sticky situations. My children have inherited my sense of humor, and I think that is a definite asset when you have TS. You have to be able to see the funny side of life.

My motor tics include eye blinking, facial grimacing, head jerking, abdominal contractions, shoulder movements, nose wriggling, tapping, lip licking, jumping, touching, smelling things, echopraxia, palipraxia, cheek biting, a big shiver that goes through my whole body, evening up things, and obsessions with symmetrical activities. My vocal tics include throat clearing, grunting, sniffing, snorting, coprolalia, echolalia, and palilalia. I have combination tics, in which I sniff, clear my throat, grimace, and move my shoulder. Most of this stuff I disguise very well.

My OCD causes a lot of strange obsessions, but the most bothersome is the fear that everyone in my family will die in a big disaster. I am a sailor, and every time I go on the boat with my family, I think we're all going to be killed. I fight the feeling and get on the boat anyway. I also am afraid to wear green and black together, and I am afraid of the number 13. I have some strange ideas regarding my relationship with God, and what will happen if I don't please Him.

I have an obsession with watching the angle of streetlights so much so that it distracts me while driving. I also used to have this overwhelming desire to open the car door when I was driving on the highway. Resisting this urge was a problem. Until I started taking meds, I was unable to drive outside of my town; I was a prisoner of my own fear. I had some problems keeping my license. Now, I drive anywhere I want.

I count everything—including my footsteps. I have to walk on any lines on the floor or ground, and if there is a pattern on the floor, I have to walk in a pattern too. I check and recheck things. I measure the relationship of all objects that I see—checking middle distance and relationship to another object—say windows to doors to tiles on the ceiling.

I also can't touch dirty things—especially animals. I wash my hands a lot, but don't like to use soap because it is dirty from other people's dirty hands. I also have to watch what fabrics I wear. I can pretty well only stand cotton. I can't stand to touch synthetics. I can't stand to touch any fabrics with my feet. Mostly I wear sandals all year. I also have to have a certain texture on my hands and fingers when I rub them together. Any contamination by soap, chemicals, or sticky things will change that texture and I won't be able to stand it. Then I will lick my fingers until I get that texture back. I also cannot stand repetitive sounds and electronic noises.

When I was diagnosed with TS and OCD, I found out there were medications that could make my life more bearable, so I started taking meds. I take Orap *(Pimozide)* and Prozac *(Fluoxetine)*. The change has been amazing. I don't take huge doses, but it has changed my life totally. The lifesaver has been the Prozac. Before I began taking medication, I used to go into a rage and cause all sorts of hurt to people, and afterwards I couldn't even remember what I said and did. I would then go into a deep depression and want to drive my car off the end of the pier or into a brick wall. Once I started taking the Prozac, I no longer wanted to do these things. The Orap has pretty much stopped the rages. I used to feel like I had this cloud inside my head that needed to explode. After the explosion, I would feel relief and the cloud would go away for awhile until the next buildup. That cloud is no longer with me. The side-effects aren't great but I am willing to live with them, because I am so much happier and content in my life. I have, however, gained sixty pounds and I have a tremor on the right side of my body. One of the possible side effects of Orap is tardive dyskinesia. If I begin to show symptoms of this condition, I will probably stop taking the Orap.

What I'm left with is manageable. I don't really care too much about my tics. I don't care if anyone thinks they make me look ugly or anything. I am what I am. I no longer hurt people the way I used to, and I am actually comfortable with people now.

My doctor believes that both my parents have TS and OCD. My father has some TS symptoms, and really bad OCD. My mother has real bad OCD and some tics. I also think my paternal grandfather had TS.

I have two sisters and four brothers. My eldest sister tells me that she counts things and fools around with the numbers on license plates in her head. My younger sister has some kind of problem—a terrible rage and arguing problem—as well as some eye blinking and eye opening tics. I believe my eldest brother has TS and OCD—he has a horrible temper, inappropriate reactions to situations and inflexibility. Two of my other brothers exhibit signs of TS and OCD; however, my youngest brother has not shown signs of either disorder.

I have two boys—aged 21 and 14. The 21-year-old has OCD, ADHD, and panic-anxiety disorder. He is in complete denial and will not take any meds prescribed for him. He thinks his brother and I are freaks. He no longer lives with us. My 14-year-old has TS, OCD, and ADHD. Up until two months ago he took Risperdal *(Risperidone)*, Prozac, and Ritalin *(Methylphenidate)*. Unfortunately, the Risperdal gave him such awful side-effects—huge weight gain, lethargy, elevated prolactin levels, and subsequent formation of breasts. As a result, the doctor suggested he stopped taking the Risperdal; I agreed. It has been quite a ride since then. He is still taking the Prozac and the Ritalin. He is so full of anger, and he is in a rage most of the time. He is abusive to my husband and me, both physically and verbally. He is like a different person. There are rare moments of peace. That is a whole story unto itself.

We knew that this child was different from the day he was born. He was born with two teeth, and immediately got into this biting habit that was very hard to break. He also had projectile vomiting, so he was not the type of baby that people wanted to pick up. In fact, I feel that that is where the isolation problem really began. By the age of two, he had terrible rage tantrums. As a parent, you expect that the "terrible twos" will one day pass, but with him it never did. He had a wonderful imagination and was always making things and dressing up in costumes he had made of some cartoon character he liked. On one occasion, my mother received a knock on the door and a man told her that there was a small boy up on the roof. He was in the Peter Pan stage, and thought as Peter Pan there was nothing wrong with being on a slippery roof in an ice storm. He was only three.

When he started school there was a big problem with separation anxiety. By the second grade there was a serious problem with school. His teacher didn't like him. In hindsight, I think she just didn't know what to do with this kind of kid. He didn't fit all the models she'd seen previously. She was mistreating him. On one occasion, she had him stand up in front of the whole class and talk into a tape recorder about all the bad things he had done during that day. On other occasions, she gave the entire class ice creams but wouldn't give him one because he was bad. When we found out about this we insisted the Principal discipline her. On another occasion, my mother arrived at the school early to pick him up and found him crying outside in the hall. Apparently, this was a regular thing for him, to be made to stand out in the hall for disrupting the class. My mother gave the teacher a piece of her mind and took my son home with her. We had several meetings with the Principal and teacher that year; however, the problems continued.

The following year, in third grade, things finally came to a head. My son had a pet iguana, and it died suddenly. He became so distraught that we kept him home from school for several days. When he returned to school, he saw a boy in the library pick up a book on iguanas. He attacked the boy. Later that day, he threw his desk at his teacher. At this point, the school insisted we take him to see a doctor. That is when the diagnosis was made. After the school and teachers found out about his diagnosis, they became much more cooperative and positive. There was still the odd time that I had to fight for his rights, and there was still the odd teacher who did not understand that he couldn't control some of his behavior. There was one teacher who abused the non-violent crisis intervention holds, for example. I found that if you join with the school and are on their side, that they will treat you with respect and give your child some slack.

There was a case last year, in ninth grade, in which my son and a supply teacher had a disagreement. The teacher sent my son to the office. He talked to the Vice-Principal and she said under the circumstances he should just wait out the class, and go at the end to pick up his books. When he returned to the class, some classmates said to him, "You should have heard what he said about you." My son approached this teacher and said, "I hear you were talking about me." This teacher said, "You are not even worth my speaking to." My son continued to pursue the issue and said, "You told the class that I was mentally ill and that I took a lot of medications. You had no right to say this. This is confidential information about me." The teacher said, "You belong in a mental hospital." My son told him he was going to report him to the office, and that he was going to be in a lot of trouble. The Vice-Principal dealt with the matter satisfactorily. The school could not fire this teacher as he had a short-term contract, but they assured me his contract would not be renewed the following month. They also assured me that my son would never have to be in a class with him again. Unfortunately, this did not happen, and my son had to spend the occasional class in the Principal's office to avoid him. This was not fair, but apparently the school was unable to rectify the situation in any other way. As I said previously, generally the school has been very cooperative and understanding of my son's problems, especially since he has gone off the meds. But, I have to always be ready to stand up for his rights if I think they've been compromised.

I have such tremendous gifts from having TS. I am an artist. I paint, draw, and have danced most of my life. I work as an Engineering Specifications Writer and my job involves checking things and looking for mistakes, and I must be extremely accurate. This suits my extreme perfectionism, but as my doctor told me-the meds will make me check things twice not ten times. On the other hand, though, I came close to being fired from my job around the time that I started my meds. I had such a bad reputation for not getting along with others, not being able to bend, and not being able to accept change, my obsession with being "perfect," and my rages. I was very difficult. I stopped being invited to meetings. No one wanted to deal with me. I also had a terrible problem with being late. The only thing that saved me was my sense of humor. Things have changed greatly since then. I think I get along with people very well now. I have been on many teams, and have even been a team leader. I think it has helped that I'm very bright and have an excellent memory, although the meds seem to dull my memory a bit.

The benefits of TS are also evident in my family. Most family members are also very artistic. My father was a photographer/journalist. My paternal grandfather was an artist/photographer. My youngest son is an artist and is musically gifted. Hopefully he will pursue these things as a career.

TWO TEACHERS' LESSONS

■ ■ ■

These lessons are not only about Tourette's; they are about acceptance, love, and compassion. I applaud Angela and Brad for choosing a profession that is so often taken for granted. After all, teachers are, next to the parents, a child's most influential role model.

EDUCATE OUR EDUCATORS

Angela C. Reinheimer

I began ticcing in the first grade. I shook my head, twitched my nose, and blinked and winked my eyes. There was an occasional utterance, but I kept those as quiet as possible so no one could hear. School was very stressful for me. I was such a mommy's girl that I was afraid to go to school for a whole day. My teacher was old, ill, and missed many classes; as a result, the school sent in substitute teachers. These subs scared me and stressed me out even more. I was a bright student and made excellent grades, but I feared school and this caused my tics to get worse. I would frequently visit the nurse and feign illness in order to go home, where I felt it was safe.

The first doctor I saw for my tics was my pediatrician. My mother was told I was just a nervous child. My parents considered this an acceptable diagnosis. By this time, I was aware that I was not normal and my friend's mom suggested that I might have Tourette syndrome (TS) because her brother had it.

I have seen many neurologists over the years. The first one made me feel like an idiot. He initially suspected TS and asked me if I ever barked like a dog. I told him I didn't. He then asked my parents if I barked or made any other kind of noise, and they also said no. He decided that I did not have TS because I didn't bark like a dog, which he mistakenly believed was the most common symptom of people with the disorder. Like my pediatrician, he concluded that I was just a nervous child. He put me on medication, but my parents kept me on them for only a short while (around a year). I believe that my parents stopped giving me the medications because my dad didn't notice any difference and said he "wasn't paying for something that didn't work."

When I was about to enter the seventh grade, my parents noticed that my tics were getting much worse. They also saw how stressed out I was about having to start a new school (junior high). They took me to the neurologist and he put me back on medication. I was given IQ tests and psychological batteries. The only test that I remember taking was the Rorschach. I had to have an EEG and blood tests, but after all of that, it was again decided that "she's just a very nervous little girl." I hated being called that. I hated not knowing why I couldn't control my eyes, nose, and head.

The neurologist I was seeing retired when I entered my sophomore year of college. I found another doctor, and he also did all the tests with the exception of the EEG. Finally, this doctor confirmed that I had a mild case of TS. He recommended that I see a psychologist in order to help me deal with my problems. I saw a psychologist twice and decided I didn't like her course of treatment. She would have me talk about my father, who was an alcoholic, and have me daily record my dreams. I told my father I wanted to stop seeing her because she upset me so. Of course, I couldn't tell him why. The medications were helping so I just decided to leave well enough alone.

My father found another neurologist, this one closer to home. I have been seeing him for the past seven years. He has a great reputation and treated the Archbishop of St. Louis when he was diagnosed with a brain tumor. He is really great. I feel very comfortable with him. I see him once a year for a checkup. He asks me how I feel, does a few quick checks on me, we chat a bit, and I'm on my merry way. He has me on Klonipin *(Clonazepam)* daily. He said when I feel stressed, I could increase the dosage. I like that he trusts me to know what is in my best interest.

As for my tics, I twitch my nose, I shake my head a little, and I blink my eyes often. Sometimes it appears that I am winking (which has gotten me into a bit of trouble at times). Occasionally, I catch myself starting to repeatedly clear my throat, but if I realize I'm doing it, I usually stop. One other thing I do constantly that is not apparent to others is popping my ears. I can hear the sound clearly in my head, and I guess it has become a common tic for me because I can do it without anyone knowing.

I believe I have had periods of obsessive-compulsive disorder and attention deficit disorder. When I was a little girl, I remember getting up after being put to bed to go to the bathroom about five or ten times in a half-hour period, something my parents didn't know. I was always afraid I would wet the bed, even though I never had. This didn't last long. One thing that I still do is check my alarm clock before I go to sleep. I may check it three or four times in a ten-minute period to make sure it is set. That's as repetitive as I get.

I have never been hyperactive, but I was always the kind of child that couldn't do one thing for long periods of time other than read or watch TV. I have my own little quirks—I love things with numbers and I have my favorite numbers that I tend to fixate on. I can't ever sit still; I'm always changing the position in which I'm sitting. I like to be in control of most things; I have been told I'm very bossy, which is probably why I make a good teacher—I get to be in control (somewhat).

My tics have remained pretty consistent over the years. I still have the three I started with. However, because my medication works well for me, and maybe because I am older, they are much less noticeable. People usually comment that they thought I just had a cute little nervous habit (what's cute about it?). Some people even argue with me when I say I have TS. A girl once accused me of lying just to try to get sympathy from people!

I think I've been pretty lucky with my TS. It really doesn't interfere with my ability to do anything I want to in my life. I function just like everyone else. It has helped me in my line of work because whenever we have a student in our school with TS, I speak to him or her and the teacher to help them understand how it affects the child. I don't think having TS has ever been an issue in anyone's life but my own and my parents'.

No one in my family has TS. My mother characterizes one of her aunts as "nervous," but there are no confirmed cases of it on either side of the family. My mother thinks that her brother's Parkinson's and my TS are related, but I don't know.

My parents had me when my mother was 40 and my father was 43. My two sisters were 16 and 18. I spent a lot of time with my middle sister growing up. She married at 19 and had her first baby at 21. Her family became my second family. I traveled with them and would spend weeks on end with them. I think she wanted me to have as normal a life as I could away from my father. My parents didn't do the Little League thing with me. If I wanted to do anything growing up, I recall it being discouraged because they didn't want to have to leave the house. This is probably because it cut into my dad's drinking time. It was very stressful in my house, and this would make my tics worse.

My father was not so understanding. He may have thought

I did it on purpose. I remember more than one occasion when he would tell me to sit still and not twitch and he would watch the clock. He would see that I could go for five minutes or more and say something to the nature of, "If you can do that now, why don't you do that all the time?" I would leave the room and my tics would just increase in intensity. He would stare at me at times and ask what was wrong. I would say nothing, and he would ask why I was shaking so badly. *Damn...it was that obvious.* My father was never violent, but there were a lot of emotional issues and he was extremely controlling; sometimes he was just verbally mean. I don't want to use the word abused, because my father has been sober now for five years, and I love him dearly. I would never want him to think he hurt me while I was growing up. I don't want to ever say emotional abuse because that, too, would hurt him; however, how do you quantify what I grew up with? I guess saying that my father was an alcoholic around whom I had to tread lightly would be sufficient. I never stirred the waters around him; I always followed the rules.

When a boyfriend pressured me to have sex, or I considered going away to college or quitting college, it was not easy to talk to my father. When I was stressed, I would go to my sister's house, where everything was easy. Up until my senior year of college, I spent most weekends at her house. Both she and my other sister were extremely understanding, as was my mother. It was never a discussion unless I wanted it to be. I don't ever remember feeling self-conscious around them. My mother used to say she wished she could take it away from me, and she would let me sit in front of her and she would rub my scalp, my neck, and my face. It was nice that she did this for me; it was soothing and helped me to relax.

At this stage in my life, my family is very understanding

about my tics. No one mentions them anymore other than my parents asking if I see my doctor, how he is doing, and what does he say about me? I remember thinking I would never have a boyfriend because he wouldn't want to kiss a face that twitched, but I have had several serious relationships where it has never been an issue.

I once had a religion teacher who would mimic me and ask why I ticced. It was humiliating because this was around the sixth or seventh grade and boys were watching! I would just sink in my chair and say, "I don't know." I don't think I ever told my parents about her, but I remember begging them weekly not to make me go to religion school. I hated her then. As I got older, when someone would ask why I did "that" (as they put it), if I felt they were just being rude, I would quickly retort, "Well, why do you _____?" and comment on some characteristic of theirs that stood out. If the person seemed sincere, I would just say I have TS and let it go at that. That seemed to be enough for most people. I remember a guy who was sitting across from me (I don't remember where I was) and he was trying to flirt with me by twitching his nose like mine, smiling, then asking why I did that. I said, "Well, I have an excuse why I do what I do, but watching you do it, knowing you have no justifiable reason, just makes you look like an ass!"

As a child, I hated that I couldn't control it. I hated that everyone could see and make fun of it. I hated how obvious and humiliating it was. I remember a kid in junior high who mimicked and teased me. He finally asked, "Why do you do that?" My response was, "I was in a car accident and I have shards of glass in my eyes and it's a constant reminder that this accident killed my parents." I ran away from him crying, hoping he felt awful. From what the group around him told me, he felt horrible for teasing me, but no one bothered to tell him I had lied about the accident because most of them knew how sensitive I was about my tics.

As an adult, I can live with TS. It doesn't affect my day-to-day life at all. I feel "normal" if there is actually a definition for normal—mine being "someone who does not have TS." This may irritate others with the disorder who do consider themselves normal, but growing up I did not feel that way at all. So when I say I feel normal, I mean I feel as if I don't have TS; it isn't present in my everyday life. But I have thought about it often lately, and I recently joined an e-mail ring—TSWorld—so I could talk to others about living with TS. My biggest concern, as I get older, is whether or not I should have children. What is the likelihood that they would inherit my disorder? I have said I wouldn't have kids; I have said I would. I toss the idea back and forth. Could I bring a child into this world knowing that he or she may have a disorder that could easily be severe? How can I go through my life not experiencing childbirth, not having a child of my own? These are the things I think about now. I really don't have to worry too much about it because I am single at this point, but I hope to be married someday and consider having a family. The other part of me says that there is no way I can have a child knowing that I could possibly give that child this disorder. It is confusing and saddening to think about.

If I could get rid of my TS, I would because I don't want to continue twitching for the rest of my life. However, today I can say I'm a good human being, a caring person and educator, most likely because I have experienced life with TS. It's a double-edged sword.

I was in a gifted art program in elementary school; I took Art in high school. My twelfth-grade drawing teacher used to beg me to become an art teacher. If I really wanted to, I could be quite good at what I do. Right now my artistic nature is focused on taking photos and doing layouts in scrapbooks using decorative paper, stickers, and colored pens. It allows me to be creative and have fun with a group of friends who are also interested in this hobby. I love to write in my journal, and in high school I wrote a lot of papers that the teachers would try to get me to enter in contests. I graduated as one of five seniors to be recognized for outstanding achievement in communication arts. I have not, however, cultivated my talents into anything further than a hobby. I think it's because I can't stay focused on one thing for long periods of time.

The thing that bothers me most is that people who do not know anything about TS assume it is the "cursing disease." When I mention that I have it, they say, "Really? You don't curse." Movies also play up TS as a cursing disease. I have seen plenty that have focused on only the most extreme aspects of the disorder, all of which seem to include shouting of expletives. It is an annoyance that these television shows and movies incorrectly educate society about TS. I can laugh at them, but it does bother me that it is stereotyped in this way. And one show that I do respect, *Seventh Heaven,* had an episode in which a young boy kept calling out in church, but I don't recall his having any noticeable tics. Again, this is not a correct representation of TS.

What advice do I have? The only thing I can say is have *patience.* Everyone around someone with this disorder, including the person with it, needs to be patient. Reduce stress in that person's life; don't add to it. Ignore their tics; don't ridicule. Realize that when the tics are extremely obvious, the person is most likely stressed. Help him or her find ways to calm down. Educate our educators! As a teacher, I have had many children who have disorders and diseases, and the parents are always quick to inform me of how to deal with that child. It helps to inform the class and school as a whole. Ignorance comes from a lack of knowledge, and ignorance breeds cruelty. If people are educated about TS, they will be more accepting.

■ ■ ■

If you would like to contact Angela, you can do so by sending her e-mail at **mookey72@aol.com.**

SALLIE MAE FIRST YEAR TEACHER OF THE YEAR

Brad Cohen

Brad was generous enough to allow me to adapt the following story from a speech he has given at various venues in the Southeast.

Tic, tic, bang, bang, tic, bang, tic, tic, bang, bang, bang, tic, bang, tic, tic, bang, bang, bang, clap, tic, clap, clap, tic, clap, clap, tic, tic, tic, clap, clap, clap.

What is a *tic?* A tic is an involuntary movement or sound that I do all day, everyday, because I have Tourette syndrome.

What is a *bang?* A bang is every time a person told me to shut up, be quiet, leave the room, stop it, or go away. It is every time a person did not believe in me; it is every person that did not and could not accept me for who I was.

What is a *clap?* A clap is every time somebody accepted me for who I was; it is every time someone helped me when I was down; it is every time that someone encouraged me to move forward, followed me in the right direction, and respected who I was.

I have had Tourette syndrome since I was seven years old and it has not been easy. As a matter of fact, it has *always* been a challenge. When you are presented with a challenge, you must decide how you will take on that challenge. Will it be a challenge that you take head-on? Or will it be a challenge that you try to avoid? I decided to take my challenge head on and not let Tourette's beat me. You see, it's like a little game of Brad Cohen versus Tourette syndrome. Whoever stands the longest will win.

I never let Tourette syndrome stand in my way. I refuse to use Tourette's as an excuse to not succeed in life. That would be too easy; Tourette's would win. If I always allowed Tourette syndrome to get the best of me, then how could I ever make a difference on others? How would I ever be able to look at myself in the mirror and be proud of who I am? I decided not to make it a game of Brad Cohen versus Tourette's; I decided to become partners with Tourette's.

Growing up all I ever wanted was to be like the other children in my class. They were normal. They didn't have tics. They didn't make noises. For me, it was an uphill battle because not many people knew what Tourette syndrome was. "Brad, would you come up here in front of class and apologize for making so many disruptions today?" So I got up out of my seat and I apologized to my fifth-grade class. "I'm sorry for making the noises; it won't happen again." My teacher smiled and told me to take a seat.

Also that year, I remember my teacher made me apologize to the class for making noises that I could not control. I don't remember the field trips, I don't remember the science experiments, but I do remember my first classroom speech.

Growing up with a disability was not easy. Teachers didn't know how to handle certain situations, so they kicked me out of class. I recall my seventh-grade teacher putting me in time-out every day because he thought I was hiccupping on purpose. He did not want to acknowledge the fact that I had Tourette syndrome, and that I could not control the noises that I was making; therefore, everyday for math I would sit across the hall. Here I was, the student that sat in the corner looking at a white wall while the rest of the class was learning something valuable. While they were learning math, I was learning how to survive in a society which did not tolerate differences. At the time, I didn't realize what a valuable lesson I *was* learning.

It was then that my inner strength took control. I constantly reflected on who I was and whether I was good enough. I learned at a young age that ignorance is bliss in our society. I needed to determine how I was going to overcome my disability while at the same time teach individuals to cope with those who are different. Taking the initiative to educate others about my condition was the role that I assumed. It was up to me to teach those around me that I was to be treated like they were treated. I knew it was important to learn as much about my disability as I could so I could educate the public. *I* had to be the expert. If I didn't understand my own disability, then how could I teach others about my condition? This was very important to me as it allowed me the opportunity to understand who I was and what I needed to do to survive the obstacles that would be placed in front of me for the rest of my life.

It all started in eighth grade when I gave a speech to the entire junior high student body educating them about Tourette syndrome. By taking this first step, I taught others to accept me for who I was. This was a pivotal point in my life. I truly matured on that day and learned that I am capable of anything as long as I put my mind to it.

I realized that ignorance could only be stopped by education. This is why I am open and honest with everyone about Tourette's. I have what I call the "one chance" rule. I am willing to give everyone at least one chance to mess up. If someone comes up to me and tells me to shut up or leave a restaurant, I explain that I have Tourette syndrome and what it is. The next move is theirs. They can either accept what I have said or they can decline it. If they believe me and understand me then I have no problem; but if they continue to harass me, that is when I get a little upset. I must realize that not everyone understands Tourette's. I must give others the benefit of the doubt because many people want to do the right thing.

My life has been a series of challenges, but each challenge has brought me closer to where I am today. Do I regret having Tourette's? No, I don't. Tourette's is now part of my personality and I would not be the same person without it. Tourette syndrome is like my best friend, in the way that it's always with me and it understands who I am. It will never leave, so I learn to get along with it. And we enjoy each other's strengths as well as weaknesses.

Sure I doubt myself and I get upset when I get kicked out of movies, restaurants, and libraries. But at the same time I realize that I can only do so much. I must pick and choose my battles. My biggest battles were often in social, family, and academic situations. Growing up, people thought I was possessed by the devil. They thought I was just a bad kid. Friends and relatives didn't want to be around me because they said my tics embarrassed them when we were out in public. In junior high I had no friends. I mean who wanted to be friends with the guy who made noises all day? If you weren't the best looking, the athlete, the most popular kid, then you were the dork or the geek or the nerd, or the kid in the corner who made noises. Who wanted to be friends with the noisemaker? I ate lunch by myself and other kids would parade around me and mock each tic that I made. Some kids would actually fight me thinking they could somehow stop these noises.

School was always difficult for me, as my teachers had a hard time understanding what was bad behavior and what was Tourette's. Well, the answer was simple to me: *most of it was Tourette's*. But the teachers didn't want to hear that, and they didn't know how to handle it when I told them. I would get poor grades and a poor education because many of the teachers could not look past the Tourette's. What was there to like about school? Being sent to the principal's office all the time? Talking to counselors all day? It wasn't until high school and college when my education actually became meaningful to me.

This is why I wanted to be a teacher. I saw so many bad things in the field of education and I knew I could fix them. Ever since I was in junior high, I knew I was going to be a teacher that would be there for those students who had disabilities and difficulties, because *I* wanted to be the role model that I never had in school. I wanted to make a difference in young children's lives and teach them that they can be whatever they want, as long as they work hard at it.

Pursuing the teaching profession was one of the easiest decisions of my life. In 1996 I graduated cum laude from Bradley University with a Bachelors degree in Education. As I walked across the graduation stage, I first thought of what a great accomplishment it was to graduate from college. Then I reflected on where I came from and the uphill battle I had overcome. I was now one step away from making a difference in children's lives.

The next step of my life was one that would test who Brad Cohen really was. It would be a step that would test any individual. I began to interview with schools throughout the Atlanta area for a teaching position. Interview after interview administrators would fire questions at me about philosophy, classroom management, discipline, lesson plans, and my background with children. My resume was flawless, showing good grades and numerous leadership experiences. My letters of recommendation were beautiful. With each interview, I got better. I became one of the best interviewees because I was getting so much practice.

Although the practice was great, I was beginning to see a distorted picture of society. My biggest fears in life were standing directly in front of me, as I was turned down one interview after another. As I left the interviews, I knew by the looks on the principals' faces that they *knew* they had a qualified candidate. But they weren't willing to take the *risk*. They weren't willing to take a *chance*. People could not look past my Tourette's and see me for who I really was. Although it was illegal, principals asked me several questions about Tourette's and my disability: "What is Tourette's? What does it cause you to do? How do you deal with it?" And I answered them. But these were not the questions that disturbed me; I expected these. The questions that really shocked me were the ones that got to the root of what the principals really wanted to know. "How will children be able to learn while you're making your noises all day in the class? How will we inform the children about Tourette's? How will we explain this to the parents? What will our faculty say? How will our community react to our hiring you?"

These people couldn't look past my Tourette's to get a clear view of me as a teacher. I realized these schools were not for me and I knew that I needed to find a school that would respect me for who I was. The school would have to accept my Tourette's *and* see my contributions to the classroom. I would not settle for anything less. It would take a special administration to see it. Was there a taker? Could anyone see past the Tourette's? I wasn't willing to give up. I've always believed that good things come to those who wait, and I knew that I had waited long enough.

On my *twenty-fifth* interview, in September of 1996, I was given the chance to be a second-grade teacher at Mountain View Elementary School. These wonderful people were able to see something that twenty-four others could not see. They were willing to take the risk and help me to succeed and be the

best teacher that I could be. They helped me get my first position as a second grade teacher. Well, I didn't have to wait long
to prepare for my new classes as school was already in session. I
jumped into the position immediately. It didn't take much time
for me to prepare because I had been prepared for this day my
whole life.

On the first day of school I got the Tourette's issue out of
the way as I educated my students. I told them that there was
something in my brain that makes me make noises and tics
that I cannot control just like there is something in their brains
that causes them to blink their eyes. I was open and honest
with them about who I was and what I might do. I allowed
them to ask as many questions as they wanted. The kids were
great and they quickly understood Tourette's. They were able
to go home and educate their parents. As a matter of fact, my
students became my biggest advocates. When kindergartners
would come up and mock me, my second graders would say,
"Don't make fun of him. He can't help it. There's something in
his brain that makes him make these noises just like there's
something in your brain that makes you blink!" Well, the
kindergartners would get this weird look on their faces, and
they would just run away, and say "Okay!"

My first year was great and I made the most out of every
opportunity. My first class was very special to me and I tried to
give them the best education possible. I gave some great lessons and I made some silly mistakes. But with each mistake, I
got better. One reason I feel I was so good my first year was
because *I was myself.* I taught people to have a sense of humor
about Tourette's. Sometimes I'd be teaching and I'd be walking
around the room looking at all the students' papers and all of a
sudden a noise would come out of my mouth, and a little kid
in front of me would pop out of his seat and say "Oh! You
scared me!" And I would say back to him, "Good!"

Sometimes I would leave the room for a second when the

kids were doing their work. Now most of the time when a teacher leaves the room, the kids get off task, but when I returned to class they were sitting in their seats working. They were angels. But then one kid told me that they would all hear me making my noises in the hall as I returned, and they would quickly get quiet and put their heads on their tables as I walked into class. I told them this is why I don't play hide-and-go-seek and we will not be playing it in our classroom!

I had some great moments with that class. But no moment would've prepared me for what happened at the end of the school year. A faculty meeting was called and I heard one of our administrators introduce a person from the county office that had a special announcement to make. This is when I found out that I had won the *Sallie Mae First Year Teacher of the Year Award* for Cobb County. I could not believe it; I was speechless. I could not believe that they thought I was the best first year teacher in the county. It was an honor. But the best was yet to come, as a few months later I went on a trip to Washington D.C. and received the *Sallie Mae First Year Teacher of the Year Award* for the *entire state of Georgia*. This was an awesome honor. What did I do to deserve this? What did other teachers *not* do to deserve this? Was I truly the best first year teacher? Well, I'm not sure if I knew the answers to these questions and I really wasn't sure I wanted to dig for them. But what I did know was that I made it. For every person that doubted me there was a group of people who believed in me.

As I accepted this award I could only think of where I had come from. I thought of the fifth-grade teacher that made me get up in front of the class and speak. I thought of my seventh-grade teacher who had always kicked me out of class. I thought of all the principals who doubted my ability to teach young children. I thought of the long interviews and the silly questions that I encountered. But I also thought of the dedication that I gave to the profession during the previous year. I thought of all of those who believed in me, and had confidence that I could be a success. I thought of my parents who supported me as I grew up. And I thought of the students who had learned from me that year. Forget math and reading and writing and science. These children learned bigger lessons in life. They learned lessons on accepting others no matter what disability they may have. They learned that if they had a disability or a weakness, they could overcome it. I wanted them to say, "If Mr. Cohen can do it, so can I."

Since my first year of teaching, I have grown as both a teacher and a person. I still make noises and tics that I can't control and I'm still happy. My philosophy in life has not changed. Tourette syndrome is not a disability, it is an opportunity. Tourette's has allowed me to make a difference with people that otherwise would not be possible. I tell others with Tourette's that they cannot choose not to have it, but they can choose to accept it. That is what I have done. Being a teacher in a classroom is only part of the role I now play in our society.

I continue to prove to people that living life to its fullest is necessary. Ever since I was a child, I dreamed of being the mascot for the St. Louis Cardinals baseball team. Fredbird was a legend in St. Louis. When the other kids would run up and get their picture taken with Fredbird, I would step back and say, "I don't want a picture with Fredbird, I want to *be* Fredbird." Years later, my dream came true when I was hired to be on the character staff for the Atlanta Braves. This part-time job during the summertime gave me a chance to be close to baseball and people while fulfilling my dream. What a great job it was, as I danced around with fans and took pictures with each one of them. If they had only known who was inside the uniform, they might have been shocked.

At the same time, Tourette syndrome has taught me to

appreciate different aspects of life. This might be the reason I have become involved with organizations like the American Cancer Society and its Relay for Life event. I know that Tourette's is a minor condition compared to the deadly illness of cancer. Because of volunteering efforts and giving back to the community, Ben and Jerry's awarded me the Citizen Cool "Golden Cone" Award. This award is given out to people who demonstrate the essence of giving back to the community. And that brings me to where we are today.

What can I tell the parents of children with Tourette's, ADHD, and OCD? I say be your child's number one advocate. Fight for your child's needs and support them. Believe in them. You need to help educate them about their condition. Be open and honest. And let them hear the truth instead of hiding the truth. Telling your child, "You have a disability," might be one of the toughest things you ever have to do. But think about your child. What if you were making noises and had tics that you couldn't control and you didn't understand it? The day I was diagnosed was one of the *happiest* days of my life. Because I was able to give my problem a name and I realized that I was not the only person out there in society with this condition. Help your child realize that he or she is normal, and that there are others who have gone through the same experiences as they are going through. It is not bad to admit a problem; it's the first step toward dealing with it. This problem will only be a problem if you make it a problem. I don't see it as a problem. I have not allowed Tourette syndrome to stand in my way; I live my life just as you do. In school, be sure to educate the administration, the teachers, and the other children. They must be prepared and you need them on your side. As for the children, they are never too young to learn about Tourette syndrome. Help educate children to make your child's life a little bit easier. There are some great books, videos, and comic books to help your child explain Tourette's to others.

What I can tell the teachers that work with kids with these conditions? *Patience. Patience. Patience. Patience.* It is what separates a poor teacher from the best teacher. It is the one characteristic that keeps so many potentially good teachers away from the field of education. For the sake of a child, hold your patience as long as you can. You must remember that these children who have Tourette's, attention deficit hyperactivity disorder, and obsessive-compulsive behaviors want to be good students. But often they can't do it because there's something in their brains that tells them not to be good. These kids need good teachers. You need to educate yourself about your student's condition. Go to a conference in your area and learn about Tourette's. Talk openly with faculty, parents, and most importantly, the child. If you have a question or concern, go ask the child; you might be surprised at his or her response. Give students space. There is nothing worse than when a child needs to tic and he or she feels crowded. ADHD kids can't sit still, so don't expect them to; it's not going to happen. Have them sit somewhere in the back of the room or toward the side so they can breathe a little. I often allow my ADHD students to get a drink of water out in the hall to help them refocus. A minute break from the class can help refocus that child for ten or fifteen more minutes. Last but not least, don't think of these kids as stupid. They are actually more perceptive than you think. They know what's up and they know the game. Give them a little extra support. What type of teacher are you? The type that teaches or the type that really makes a difference? These are the students who need you most. Help them out and give them the most meaningful education you can and make a difference in their lives. *You owe them that.*

And what do I say to the children and adults who have Tourette syndrome? My Tourette's is really not so bad—it could be worse. So, I don't get to see movies when they first come out in the movie theaters, but at least I don't make my noises when I'm sleeping. I think you have to stick up for what you believe in. You have to know yourself better than anyone else. I say be open and honest and educate everyone around you. You owe it to the next person that might come around with Tourette's. Hopefully soon everyone will understand what Tourette syndrome is and it'll make all of our lives a little bit easier.

I say have a sense of humor and if you can laugh about it, people around you will feel more comfortable. Make life a little easier on yourself and try to laugh at least once a day. I also say don't use it as an excuse; that is the easy way out. Sympathy is a lousy excuse as a friend. Don't let your disability stand in your way of doing something special. Everyone has some sort of disability, but everyone has good qualities, too. Show the good qualities and let your disabilities stand as just a backdrop.

I stand before you today not looking for a sympathy vote. You can save that for somebody who really needs it. I stand here asking you to carry on my message for the many people who can't stand up for themselves. Go out there and make a difference for them. I try to make a difference every day. Now you can help me in my pursuit.

DELAYED DIAGNOSIS

■ ■ ■

Although early diagnosis of Tourette syndrome is becoming more common, there are still many individuals who live their lives in a state of self-doubt. The following stories prove that a delayed diagnosis is better than no diagnosis at all.

UP CLOSE AND PERSONAL

Michael G. DeFilippo

I am standing on the balcony of my fifth-floor hotel room in Destin, Florida, smoking a cigarette. It is five o'clock on the afternoon of July 6, 2000. I have just returned from enjoying the surf with my wife, son, and in-laws; it is a family vacation. The others are getting ready for dinner at a local restaurant.

The wind is heavy, with the heat from the parking lot rising past me. In the distance, folks are watching a young man bungee jump, children are riding a Ferris wheel, and teenagers are shuffling along the main thoroughfare carrying bags of snorkeling equipment, beach towels, and wearing colorful visors. Cars are pulling in and out of the parking lot below.

But I barely feel the wind and I am not interested in the vacationers. My sight is fixed on a spot five stories below, just beyond where the grassy island ends, and the black, steaming asphalt begins. I am wondering, *if I jumped, would I land on my feet?* The urge to do so is overwhelming; the constant desire to grab the brown railing with my hands, to feel my body as it moves up, over, and out, through the hot, sticky air, and finally, to watch the pavement as it rushes up to meet me. I continue to stare at my spot. I finish the cigarette and drop it into a small Dixie cup half-filled with water. The spell is broken. I open the door and enter the room. "Your turn for the shower, Hon," my wife calls to me from the bathroom. "Okay, here I come," I say, as I grab my evening clothes and head for the bathroom.

■ ■ ■

I grew up in the Bronx, one of the five boroughs of New York City. In school I was laughed at, ridiculed; I didn't have many friends. The few friends I did have, mostly neighborhood kids, never seemed to mention my tics. My father never let me play organized sports, his biggest reason being that I would probably just get hurt. Of course, this didn't help what little self-confidence I had to begin with.

In the sixties and seventies, New York City was a place where teenagers played stickball and handball in school play-grounds, and punchball in the streets. It didn't matter how strange you were; everyone got a chance to play. As much as I regret not having played in Little League, I am grateful for the fact that I was allowed to participate in these pickup games.

My lack of self-confidence also affected my ability to date girls. I was a late bloomer, having not experienced my first kiss until the age of sixteen. I found it difficult to approach girls because of my tics; however, in my late teens and early twenties, I had no problems dating.

My parents, sister, and relatives would tell me to stop what I was doing. Sometimes, when I went to a cousin's house, my aunt and uncle would remark that I had a "new habit" that week. Because my tics would change from time to time, new ones replacing old ones, this was a source of interest to them, I suppose.

My father was the most vocal about it, especially when we were eating dinner at a restaurant. He would tell me to stop twitching because I was embarrassing him. Of course, he didn't know that I couldn't stop the tics. At that time, even I didn't know that I couldn't control my behavior.

Today, I have integrated my tics into my daily routine and my personality to the point where they are barely noticeable. I have told acquaintances that I have Tourette syndrome (TS) and many admitted never having seen me tic, or didn't think it was anything more than part of who I am.

Even more daunting than my Tourettic tics is something that others cannot see: the intrusive thoughts that are a result of my obsessive-compulsive disorder (OCD). I do not remember having intrusive thoughts as a child or even as a teenager. I believe they started in my early thirties. The thoughts are frequent enough to cause me discomfort and make me unable to concentrate on the task at hand, and they seem to be increasing in frequency as I get older.

My thoughts involve a whole host of scenarios, from violence to sexual fantasies. My thoughts that involve sexual fantasies are not of the arousing type; I just need to go through a particular scenario in order to work through the thought.

While driving, I have also thought about driving my car across the yellow line into oncoming traffic. I have a difficult time cleaning fragile wineglasses by hand as I am seized by a compulsion to see how tightly I can squeeze them before they will break.

I have spoken with a couple of the contributors to this book who also have similar intrusive thoughts, so, I confess that I feel much better about myself, knowing that I am not the only one having these, often quite horrible, thoughts. Similarly, I am sure that these folks also feel better knowing there is someone else who experiences the same thing.

One of the most frustrating parts of my disorder is my tendency toward rage. I can blow up at the most inconsequential event, yet let more serious situations go by without much concern. I am most fearful for my son as I was raised by a father who screamed incessantly, and I do not want my son exposed to this type of behavior. I am confident that my rage is attributable to both TS and my upbringing; after all, I am a product of my past. However, I must, as an adult and a newly divorced dad, take responsibility for my actions. I must teach my son by example.

For years I wondered what was wrong with me. Every morning, I would wake up and promise myself that I would not tic anymore. I am an adult, so why should I be jerking my head the way that I do? I will just stop. Well, there is no way to *just stop*. After I learned about TS, I realized that I was tremendously foolish, yet justified, in thinking that I could stop.

I was diagnosed with TS at the age of forty. As a result of my diagnosis, I also discovered that OCD and attention deficit disorder have been, and still are, responsible for many of the other little things I do that do not neatly fall within the definition of TS. I find it amazing that I have lived with TS just about all of my life without knowing what it was; it was my worst enemy, yet my closest friend. And for thirty-three years, I didn't know its name.

Because no one knew why I ticced, I never took any medications for my symptoms. When I was diagnosed I did look into taking something for my anger. The doctor who diagnosed me offered some suggestions, but I decided that the possible side-effects far outweighed the benefits of taking these medications. I started taking St. John's Wort, an herbal mood enhancer, to see if it would help to control my anger. When I take it regularly, it does give me some time between the trigger, the event that causes the anger, and my acting out. This gives me time to decide if my reaction is warranted and also allows me to think about the consequences of my actions. In addition to St. John's Wort, I am currently taking a vitamin B complex, magnesium, calcium, zinc, vitamin C, Kava Kava, flaxseed oil, a Ginkgo Biloba supplement that includes Capsicum, Gotu Kola, and vitamin E. This combination of nutritional supplements reduces my vocal tics considerably and lessens the severity of several of my motor tics. I sometimes take Valerian Root before bedtime as it helps to calm me and reduces the tics that often accompany fatigue. If I were taking prescription medication, I would discuss these supplements with my doctor since some drugs occasionally interact with certain herbs.

I now wear a Medic Alert bracelet because I have TS, sleep apnea, am allergic to penicillin, and have a couple of food allergies. The bracelet inevitably turns a conversation to TS. When informed that I have it, many people say, "But I never heard you shout obscenities." This is the perfect opportunity for me to educate my friend or new acquaintance about TS.

I would like to tell you about a very special person. After my divorce but before I began my nutritional supplements, I was seeing a young lady who had an amazing ability to bring a peace to my life unlike any I have ever known. I believe that one's environment can play an important role in the severity and frequency of one's tics. At times of high stress, I know that my tics do worsen. I can also hold back my tics during a particular situation, say, a job interview. But this is due to a conscious effort not to tic; consequently, when I leave the interview I must release all of those tics that I held back. But what I do not understand is how during evenings spent with Laura, not only didn't I tic, but I did not have even the slightest urge to do so. I was not holding back; they were just gone. I also noticed that I never had an urge to smoke a cigarette while I was with her, and I can be a heavy smoker. I even refrained from lighting up after eating dinner at a restaurant.

Laura herself had remarked that she saw a difference in me in the first twenty minutes or so after I arrived at her place.

Initially, she said she saw some nervousness, a few tics, but everything about me changed afterward. My speech became calmer, my body relaxed and became more fluid, and my tics disappeared.

I know that I still had my chemical imbalance when I was with her. I know that my TS lay dormant, waiting for the ride home. But how could one person, by the touch of her hand, remove what had been a part of my life for thirty-six years, albeit if only for several hours at a time? I do not have that answer. But I do know this: I will never forget Laura and how my body and mind reacted when we were together. Unfortunately, our time together lasted only several weeks. It was a beautiful experience, and I must admit that there are times that I still find myself wanting to be near her, if for no other reason than to experience just one more time that life-changing sense of freedom. I only hope that everyone with TS can find his or her Laura.

■ ■ ■

If you would like to contact Michael, he may be reached at **mike@secondchancepublishing.com.**

THE BUSINESS OF LIVING

Kathryn A. Taubert

I was 38 when I finally got to say, "I was right." I loved it, even though the people to whom I might have said it were long gone from my life by then. I had no idea where they were, nor did it really matter anymore. I had always known the day would come. Being right about *It* was good enough for me. It felt good to think it anyway, if only for the old ghosts still taking up space somewhere in the back of my mind.

I was seven when *It* started: the eye blinking, head shaking, and shoulder shrugging. Soon came the accompanying grunts and whimpers, descending like rain or thunder, out of everywhere and nowhere, to confound and frighten my family and me. Those were the early years. Eventual trips to doctors resulted in little but long hours in waiting rooms, penetrating gazes, and mysterious examinations. Graduating to months of medical experimentation, these early procedures took their toll on my small, out-of-control body, only just entering its first tentative years of self-consciousness.

Life in the diagnostic dark ages of Tourette syndrome (TS) was a mixture of blessings and tortures. I now know that I was one of the more fortunate. Blessed with parents who did the best with the tools they had, I always knew their unconditional love included *It* and all the symptoms that were merely a part of me; other people were not so kind. And after the failed attempts at medicating *It* away, we dispensed with the drugs and long hours in doctors' offices, and just went on about the business of living.

My "nervous habits" were, however, long to be a mystery. Although I eventually learned how to manage them so well that most people never realized I had them, my search for answers remained with me. I believe, now, that the search led me to a thirst for knowledge that remains a part of me today. It guided my interest in biology and medicine, anthropology, and human and animal behavior. I knew that someday I would find validation for what I felt in my heart. I would find the data that proved I was not "crazy." I knew I did not feel especially nervous, disturbed, or in any other way mentally or emotionally deficient. I was bright, shy, introspective, and definitely a late bloomer.

Junior high school was hardest. Kids, jostled about the hierarchy at that age, are clearly segregated by differences into the "haves" and "have-nots." My "differences" were still pretty obvious. Although kids were relatively kinder in those days it seems, I do recall moments of depressed isolation as one of the "have-nots." I was taunted and teased from time to time, and words like "crazy" and "shaky" still bring back painful memories. Life wasn't always nice, but then it's always that way for those who are different.

My grades were quite good in everything except handwriting and advanced math. In those days, there was no special education. We had "extra work" and tutors, or we flunked and took it over again. Some students just dropped out of school, maybe to try again later.

In my case, a tutor helped me barely pass Geometry. There was, however, nothing to help my handwriting. The typewriter that would one day give rise to liberation-by-computer, was a cumbersome, frustrating tool. Nevertheless, I learned to type while struggling to have others read my handwriting. Eventually, I learned to beat the typewriter into submission until it yielded the legible paper I simply could not produce in any other way.

My social life was minimal until I was a senior in high school. My self-esteem, however, was firmly grounded by my parents' love, indulgence in music lessons, drama club, books, the family farm, a few friends, and my beloved animal companions. At the farm, I escaped into a world every child should know. My best friend, a beautiful Paint horse with whom I shared my most wonderful dreams and private torments, carried me through many long years of sometimes-social solitary confinement. These things transformed what might have been a more painful life for my twitchy body, and, I believe, helped secure my future as well.

Throughout adolescence and young adulthood, I pursued my education, marriage, and a career, but always that search continued. Driven by some need for vindication for both my parents and myself, I read everything that might lead me to the answer. In the meantime, I achieved all that I wanted in my work. An early marriage, although it did not last, did not deter me from a happier union in years to come. I achieved a satisfying career, good friends, and accomplished much for which I am proud. I learned to believe that my "condition" was in large part responsible for shaping the person I am. Although I am still a work in progress, I am content.

My late father-in-law and I shared a love of science, leading to a subscription to a science magazine. After waiting for years for the pot to boil, I eventually gave up the active search and just continued with life until that day in 1984 when *It* appeared in print. The list of symptoms for the "bizarre neurological condition" leapt at me from a remote corner of the page, staggering me with revelation.

Tourette syndrome: the name for which I had searched for more than 30 years. The identity of the *It* that gave me the right to say "I was right!" It was not a "conversion reaction," "repressed psychological conflict," or mysterious mental malady the result of some "physical or psychic trauma." *It* was biological!

In one swift moment, an immense and surprising relief overtook me. My parents were vindicated, and I was extraordinarily relieved. I knew it was not something they had "done to me," as had been implied to them so many years ago. All those years of silent searching swept away in one brief, enlightened moment. Just as I had stopped watching for the pot to boil, it did.

I had crafted a good life for myself. With the help of that foundation of unconditional love and security provided by my parents, and those teachers who saw beneath the odd mannerisms to the adult I could become, I navigated the adolescent gauntlet with my self-esteem mostly intact. In the framework of now, I think that my experience with TS taught me a lot about life, people, and especially self.

Would I change it all, knowing what I know now? TS made me who I am. I like the person I have become. It has taught me a lot. I wouldn't take any "magic pill" to make TS disappear until you could convince me that the only thing I would lose is my inability to sit still. I am not so sure now I want to be "cured" anyway!

TS did, indeed, interfere with my life in a meaningful way. I turned my emotional pain and isolation into music and writing, and from work as a professional jazz singer, I helped pay my way through college. From my early experiences overcoming obstacles, I learned problem-solving skills that led to a successful career in business.

TS influenced my social relationships, but considering the fact that good relationships are built upon much more important things than "symptoms," I cannot say that is all bad. Being shy and reserved is not exclusive to having TS. And learning to appreciate friends for who they are and not what they have is, in my humble opinion, a benefit of having TS.

I went on to get a formal diagnosis of moderately severe TS. I tic approximately 30,000 times a day. I have more than 30 different kinds of simple and complex tics, an exaggerated startle response, dysgraphia, and some relatively mild obsessive-compulsive traits. I have also suffered depression. My tics decreased in forcefulness and intensity as I matured, but, ironically, increased in frequency and number. I have never known a moment, since those early years, when I haven't ticced many times every hour, every waking moment.

I do not have first-degree relatives with TS, although the presence of other conditions often accompanying TS are evident. I have a distant relative with relatively mild symptoms of TS that was never formally diagnosed. I do not take medications, having found side-effects of those presently used for treatment to be worse, for me, than TS. I do watch my diet and exercise. I am careful to get the rest I need, which is considerable, and I have learned to assert my needs when my body tells me. I do not apologize for my differences now; I applaud them. After trying to hide *It* for 30 years, I now use every opportunity I have to discuss *It*. The dimensions of my condition have changed. Although still segregated to some extent by *It*, I am now one of the "haves." My condition is now the subject of enlightenment rather than mystery and shame.

I might want a diagnosis sooner, but only under the condition that the misinformation that often accompanies current TS information be eliminated. Parents today are burdened by too many stigmas, speculation about the condition, which has no basis in fact, and sensationalistic presentations of TS that cause a different kind of damage than I faced in the '50s. Without a diagnosis, without the hope of a "cure," we simply went on with life.

The advice I have for parents of children with TS is the same as that for parents of kids without TS. They are your children. They need the same things other children need. Perhaps more of some things and less of others, but the same things, nevertheless.

Do not think of TS as a disorder with a kid attached. Never forget that they are still kids who just happen to have a condition called TS. They are still your children. Love them. It most often is just that simple. Not having children of my own had less to do with TS than it did with a thriving career and a peripatetic nature. Admittedly, while I was one of the lucky ones, I cannot help but believe that my sometimes-painful experiences with the childhood realities of being unattractively "different" did have some influence over my decision to pursue a career instead of a family. I subsequently married into a grown family that allowed me to go straight to grandchildren. That worked for me and I have no regrets.

Yes, I would recommend that people with TS have children, if they wish. Who better to parent kids with TS than those with experience? Career aspirations notwithstanding, I get along famously with kids and animals!

TS can certainly be a disability. Most often, however, it has less to do with our symptoms than with societal attitudes. There are serious cases in which physical pain and damage can and do occur as a result of severe tics. For those of my colleagues who suffer this way, I wish there were better treatments. For most of us, however, the only treatment required is an antidote to ignorance.

I am 54 years old. I am retired from a successful career as a management consultant and organizational development specialist for a major international insurance and financial services company. I am happily married to a retired commercial airline pilot. We have family we love, and many friends and acquaintances. Everyone seems so habituated to my tics that they have virtually forgotten about them!

For those of you hoping for words of comfort, most people with TS are not disabled in any sense of the word, except by the prejudice of others. Even those of us with more severe cases can and do live very successful and fulfilling lives.

TS is not fatal, degenerative, or contagious. It is not a disease. Symptoms most often improve through the teen years. It rarely is severe enough to warrant significant medical intervention. Interestingly, there is mounting evidence that having it may also confer benefits.*

I've grown accustomed to my TS. You get used to it. In time, you may even learn to appreciate it and get on with the business of living. I did and so can you!

■ ■ ■

You can send Kathryn e-mail at **kataubert@prodigy.net.**

---

*"Functional Asymmetries in the Movement Kinematics of Patients with Tourette's Syndrome," N. Georgiou, J. Bradshaw, J.G. Phillips, R. Cunnington, M. Rogers, Journal of Neurology, Neurosurgery, and Psychiatry, 1997 63:188-195.

"Behavioral Laterality in Individuals with Gilles de la Tourette's Syndrome and Basal Ganglia Alternations, A Preliminary Report," Biol. Psychiatry 38:386-390. M.Y. Yazgan, B. Peterson, B.E. Wexler, J. Leckman, 1995.

"Tourette's Syndrome and Creativity," Oliver Sacks, British Medical Journal, 12/92.

"Fits and Starts," The Sciences, November/December 1999, Steven C. Schlozman. Abdul-Rauf deftly incorporates tics into his style: and a touch of OCD, a syndrome related to Tourette's Syndrome: Tics, Obsessions, Compulsions: Developmental Psychopathology and Clinical Care, edited by James Leckman and Donald Cohen.

LEARN, UNDERSTAND, AND ACCEPT

Leonard William Misner

Having Tourette syndrome (TS) has given me the opportunity to help others, and helping people is an awesome feeling. I have had people from all over the world come to me for advice and it feels great to be able to help in any way, even if they just need someone to talk to. Being diagnosed can be a scary thing, so I am glad to help anyone through the transition and let them know that there is a world of us out there.

I learned about my TS when a customer approached me and asked what medication I was taking for my TS. I was extremely upset because I associated TS with what I saw on television, and I knew I wasn't like that. When I got home that night I saw a television commercial. In the commercial was the outline of a man who was ticcing. I thought to myself, I do those things. At the bottom of the screen, were the words, "West Michigan Tourette Syndrome Association." I fully believe it was a sign. That was one of the best days of my life. When I was diagnosed with TS, obsessive-compulsive disorder, and attention deficit hyperactivity disorder, it felt as if ten thousand pounds of weight were lifted from my shoulders. I now had a name for the strange behavior that had haunted me since I was seven years old: *I have Tourette syndrome.*

My tics are mild to moderate and seem to be increasing with time. I shake my head, I twitch my wrists, and I strain the muscles in my neck, arms, shoulders, back, and legs. I have a tendency to touch things a lot. I also make an "f" sound and push it out so it is like a long "f." Sometimes the word "fuck" comes out, but I can keep it to a low mumble. During my time in the Marines my tics vanished, but they returned when I was discharged. I have at times injured myself by pulling muscles in my neck and back. From time to time I also hit myself in the crotch.

For me, medication has caused more harm than good. I have taken Catapres *(Clonodine)*, which stopped working after two weeks, and Tenex *(Guanfacine)*, which lowered my blood pressure to such an extent that I would almost pass out. Currently I do not take any meds.

My family is great, though it wasn't always that way. Before I was diagnosed the remarks were "What's wrong with you? Stop That!" When I was diagnosed there was a little denial by some members of my family. Now there is total support. My family is proud of the things I have done in the Tourette community and of my dedication to help. When I was asked to speak at the Tourette Syndrome National Convention in 2000, my father paid for my wife, Beth, to go with me to Washington. My wife is my biggest supporter and my best friend.

I believe that TS is responsible for my high IQ and my musical talent. I learned to play guitar and piano without the benefit of lessons; I also write songs. I have talked to blind people who have said that the loss of sight has increased all of their other senses. Maybe the thing in my brain that causes TS also enhances my creativity. My sense of humor always helped me through rough times. When I was younger I was the class clown. It made people focus more on my ability to make them laugh than on my tics.

My TS diagnosis has also stabilized my work life. I was never able to stay at a job for very long; I have been in my current job for two years now, and do not have any intentions of leaving.

Remember that television commercial that changed my life? Well, I am now the President of the West Michigan Tourette Syndrome Association and my wife is the chapter Secretary.

For those of you with TS I say feel good about yourself. If you let yourself be held down by what others say, you are destined to a life of disappointment and emotional pain. If you follow your dreams and let no one hold you down, then you will find that you can do anything you put your mind to. I have accomplished my dreams and so can you. If people around you don't understand TS, then educate them. If they still react negatively, then I guess they are the truly disabled.

■ ■ ■

You can contact Leonard at **journeyhome@webtv.net.**
Leonard's Web site is accessible at **www.angelfire.com/mi2/tourette.**

THANK YOU, DATELINE

Eric Daily

My diagnosis came as a direct result of an October, 1998 episode of Dateline NBC about Tourette syndrome (TS). So much of what was discussed caused my wife and I to begin considering the possibility that I had this disorder. Sometime later, a friend gave us some information he obtained from a TS Web site. The symptoms that we read about so mirrored my own, we pretty much self-diagnosed TS as the reason for my ticcing. But accepting that you have a disorder is not easy. Although all the pieces fit, I remained in denial until a neurologist gave us the official diagnosis. I was thirty-two years old.

I first remember ticcing as a pre-teen. My range of motor tics include abdominal jerking, eye blinking, eye rolling, squinting, facial contortions, foot dragging, foot shaking, foot tapping, grimacing, hair tossing, head jerking, shrugging, hitting, scratching, shivering, smelling things, and stepping backwards.

My vocal tics are as numerous as my motor tics: belching, grunting, guttural sounds, hiccupping, hissing, honking, puffing, screaming, sniffing, squeaking, squealing, barely audible muttering, laughing, repeating words and parts of words, repeating phrases, stuttering, throat clearing, and yelping.

When I was younger, my family was always at me to stop ticcing. My mother used to tell me to stop making those noises, and to stop blowing and puffing through my nose. I couldn't stop, and I did not know why. My mother thought I just had a nervous habit. Now, they all accept it and ignore my tics. My wife is especially supportive.

I remember that when I got married, my wife and her mother mentioned that they noticed I had some strange habits and nervous twitches, like excessive blinking and humming. I was also a compulsive cleaner, even more so with housework. And I was very methodical and systematic about how things should be done.

Before I was diagnosed I had some embarrassing situations at work. A coworker once caught me brushing my thigh every time I would do something. He mimicked me and made fun of me. I was embarrassed by this situation and I thought he was rude. I have also had coworkers stare at me, talk about me, point their fingers at me, and ask me if I'm okay. My tics all but disappeared during the five years I spent in the United States Navy.

After my diagnosis, I did some investigating into my family history. I discovered that a first cousin on my Dad's side has a severe case of TS.

I have tried two medications to relieve my tics, Catapres *(Clonodine)* and Risperdal *(Risperidone)*. Initially, the Catapres helped a little; the Risperdal helped even more. But the side-effects were awful. The Catapres caused heart palpitations, chest pains and pressure, and dizziness. The Risperdal made me nauseated and nervous, caused panic attacks, and I suffered mental and physical fatigue to such an extent that it sent me into a clinical depression. I am not currently on any prescription medications. I recently quit smoking, and looking back, I can honestly say that the nicotine helped to suppress some of my tics.

I am currently taking a self-prescribed vitamin therapy, consisting of a vitamin B-complex, a calcium, magnesium, and zinc complex, flaxseed oil, and Kava-Kava. The B-complex is an anti-stress formula, the calcium/magnesium/zinc complex is good for the nervous system, the flaxseed oil is high in Omega 3, an essential fatty acid that helps to improve cell function, and the Kava Kava is for calmness and well being. This regimen is working for me. My tics are not totally gone, but they are considerably reduced. I believe that the overall effect of this therapy is helping to reduce the stress in my life, and as a result, my tics decrease.

■ ■ ■

Eric is the founder of the Yahoo group Christians with Tourette Syndrome. You can access them at **groups.yahoo.com/group/cw_ts.**

ANOTHER WAY OF BEING

Colleen Wang

My "introduction" to Tourette syndrome (TS) came when we unknowingly adopted a son with the disorder. He began to have symptoms when he was three; he was seven when diagnosed.

I remember clearly when the psychologist suggested he might have TS. I said, "Oh no...he just has allergies." When I left the office, I did not rush to the medical library to find out about TS. I vaguely remembered a magazine article I had read years before about TS. The article had made the sufferers sound like monsters, and I remember being very disturbed by it.

My family is still shocked that I did not go to that library to find out more. I am more than a little compulsive about researching relevant medical material on problems that affect our family. So how could I let the memory of an old magazine article stop me? I think I just dismissed it out of hand...my son was not a "monster."

After my son's diagnosis was a reality, my attitude needed a major readjustment. I decided the best way to accomplish this was to find out everything I could about this disorder.

I soaked up just about everything written on TS. I read

neurology textbooks (old and new). I searched for literature on the subject. I retrieved and read all published national and international scientific papers on TS. Several of these papers were not in English, but much to my delight, I found that the library I was working with would provide me with a translated version.

None of this seemed the least bit excessive. I was just satisfying my "need to know" all there was to know so I could help my son. I learned about sensory integration difficulties, learning disabilities, behavioral, attention, and organizational difficulties, and processing problems. I talked with psychologists, psychiatrists, educators, language therapists, and anyone else that I thought might possibly have information I needed.

This was wonderful, insightful, stimulating, and very rewarding. I got wonderful strokes for "being such a good mommy." Not that my son was any better off—but at least no one thought it could be my fault. I mean—after all, look what I had been up to! I became so knowledgeable that I began to find a few "symptoms" in myself. It became a standing joke between me and my husband: when he would walk into our bedroom and find me watching TV to my usual "curl-uncurl" toe routine. *Oh, you don't have Tourette syndrome!* Hardly evidence of TS, we would agree!

By this time the new research was beginning to point toward the theory I called "Lumping and Splitting." The "Lumpers" would classify all the tic phenomena as one disorder and call all tic disorders a spectrum disorder caused by one gene. The "Splitters" would classify all tic syndromes separately considering each to be a unique phenomenon. I was often reminded of people eating. You know, the ones who pick at each food item separately and the ones who mash them all together. I found myself convinced, without reservation, by the "Lumpers." Why?

Then came my epiphany. It came in one simple toss of the head, performed by my son—you know, the *adopted* one. He had never done that particular toss before! Wow! That humble toss triggered a flood of memories. I had read about some simple occurrence triggering memory, but had never really experienced it. What a shock! I was remembering my brother. He has been dead for 23 years. *He tossed his head like that all the time.* "Oh, my God!" I was swamped with memories. He also blinked his eyes, squinted his eyes, drooped one eye, sniffed, snorted, shrugged one shoulder, lined up his toys, straightened his room, ordered his life, was the biggest pain in the neck—alive or dead—argued, fought, lied, ran away, contended, provoked, obsessed on violence—particularly hanging—what fear he had of that...until he finally hanged himself.

"Oh, my God," was all I could think! I called my mom and asked her if she remembered my brother doing any of these things. She knew about TS. Goodness knows, I had told her often enough about every facet of TS. She would know...right? *Wrong!* Oh, she remembered his movements all right and added a few more. "But those things were just his habits," she explained. Next came my dad. He remembered even more "habits" and he remembered that they got worse when he was eight years old. I was back to "Oh, my God!"

Now, as if for the first time, a puzzle began falling together. No wonder this disorder made so much sense to me.

It was about this time that I remembered listening to Dr. Oliver Sacks talk about TS and hearing his remark about TS as just "...another way of being." I really liked that attitude. It seemed so right. I had read and experienced TS with my child and perhaps my brother, but I now know I have more than a secondhand look at TS. I think the reason it took me so long to come to this realization was that none of the books and none of the articles had ever described *me*. TS has not been a major problem for me. In fact, those characteristics I attribute in part to TS are such an integral part of me that I would not want to be without them. They are woven throughout my personality and integrated into the perceptions of my reality. In many ways they have added to my life.

My childhood home was what we have come to call today "a very dysfunctional home." We moved a lot. We children went off to different schools each year. There was a significant amount of abuse at home. In fact, our home was so out of control, I looked perfect. The key word here is "perfect."

I never remember turning in a single assignment at school that had a crossed-out word or an erased number. I did the whole assignment, over and over. Three times in fact. First for "content," second for "practice," and third for "real." It became quite a problem when I went into nursing. I found my nursing notes to be like legal documents. Nothing could be erased or removed. *I had to leave it there the very first time....ugh!* I learned to organize myself before I began. (I did the first copy for content and the second copy for practice in my head!) My crossouts were some of the neatest in the history of charting. I still laugh because my efforts did not go unnoticed. They were always cited as examples of desirable charting. They were held up to student nurses as something to be emulated. I chuckle when I think of what those instructors would have had to say if they'd only known my secret. Thank God for spellcheckers and word processors!

I was an angry kid. No one complained. Compared to my brother, I still looked good. I had reason to be angry, after all. Anger didn't interfere too much with outside relationships because I wasn't so angry there, but it definitely protected me at home. It kept me separate, pulled away from the fray. In many ways, it was my salvation. Without it I would never have had the courage to put a stop to what was going on around me.

While it helped me then, it didn't just disappear. I learned to channel my anger into more productive outlets. I am a magnificent campaigner! Convince me something is bad and that it needs to be changed, and I will move mountains. I'm convinced a large number of crusaders carry a lot of generalized anger and use it to get what they want.

As an adult, someone close to me told me to "just quit being angry." I remember being quite taken aback. Anger was and is a part of me—I needed it then and I still do. Fortunately, I was able to explain the reasons why I held on to my anger so that she and I are still close friends.

I was a mouthy kid. Boy, what a mouth! I never used profanity, at least not out loud, but what I had to say, and the way I had to say it, was most impressive. My father was a teacher at my school. In fact, he was my teacher for over three years. My mouth and his teaching—what a combination! I distinctly remember overhearing teachers and many others asking my parents why they allowed me to speak to them in that manner—as if they could have made me stop! I cringe these days when I hear the same tone and provocative words coming from my son. I, too, am frequently asked why I put up with it. Well, I can kill the kid or I can keep him. There are really no other options. I keep plugging away, and so far I am electing to keep the kid.

I was a provocative teen. I remember in class in high school one day, another student leaned over and asked me something. When I answered her question, the teacher stalked back to my seat and screamed, "I told you not to talk..." and stabbed me in the head with a lead pencil. I was properly horrified; the poor teacher was fired. In retrospect, after having a child with TS, I pause and consider that I probably orchestrated the event quite nicely. Need I say, I made the most of the moment?

I recall being a very talkative kid. I have looked through my old report cards to see if my memories are correct. I found them not only correct, but understated. "Yak, Yak, Yak," that's all my teachers reported. Nothing really slowed me down. I would be moved to another part of the room when the "fun" got out of control. Moving never bothered me—I just moved the "fun" on over with me.

I would talk impulsively, but I never looked at it as something "wrong." I made a lot of friends. I nearly always smiled when I yakked, so to me it didn't seem a problem. The only real time I found my impulsive talking a problem was when the class was planning a surprise party for one of my classmates. The child involved kept asking all of us in the classroom what was up. It truly seemed a power beyond my control made the answer pop out. This did not make me a popular person for quite a while. Sigh. I was given plenty of time to repent.

While I was impulsive and talkative, I was also compulsively neat and complete. I guess the teachers liked neatness more than they disliked yakking and I got great grades.

I was a spontaneous kid and always up for a good time. I generally had enough common sense so I seldom got in over my head. I was an intense kid. It was practiced wisdom in our house not to "get me going." I never let go. I still don't. No one ever needed to steer me into assertiveness training courses. As a matter of fact, I think I could teach those techniques. I have found this characteristic to be an asset. I far prefer it to the alternative.

As I come into the present, I find that what held true as a child remains true today. I find it difficult to know whether these characteristics stem from TS or are part of some "other" part of me. I do know that many of the people I meet that have TS share many of these characteristics. Are they part of TS or part of us? Who knows? I think the reality is it doesn't really matter. But I'm getting ahead of myself now.

A few years ago, I began taking medication for an endocrine (hormone) disorder. One of the medications I was taking was Buspar *(Buspirone)*. I realized that it had begun to be a problem for me. I found I had become depressed and "stuck." I would ruminate on a problem without result for hours, never coming to any conclusion. I felt like I was curling inward. My husband would find me just sitting frozen in our bedroom. He was very concerned and would ask me what was wrong. To which I answered "nothing...I'm just thinking."

In desperation I tried some of my son's Anafranil *(Clomipramine)*. This gave me function. I was not, however, "fixed." When I described these difficulties to my physician he withdrew me from Buspar and recommended I take Wellbutrin *(Bupropion)*. My reaction was ridiculous. I refused, saying "I can't take that! My son takes that for TS!" *I didn't have Tourette syndrome!* But I was willing to take Anafranil, which he also took for TS and obsessive-compulsive disorder. Go figure.

After I was told I had been showing early signs of a pseudo-Parkinson's, I quit being ridiculous and started the Wellbutrin. What a relief. I had an almost total reversal of depression symptoms and complete relief from headaches. With the relief I gained I was able to begin looking seriously at my "other symptoms."

There was a lot more to look at than my "curl-uncurl" toe trick. I had always driven people crazy with repetitious finger-nail piano tapping. I also regularly jiggled my legs and feet. I would click and unclick pens, flash a high five while holding the steering wheel when driving a car. Mind you, none of these were really a problem. In fact, almost no one except me knew that I did them. I had rarely paid them notice. I hadn't tapped around any one person enough to be noticed for years.

I am compulsively neat and organized. I guess I didn't

really understand how neat until I called an old college room-mate while visiting Atlanta. I angled for an invitation to visit, and after meeting for dinner in a restaurant, I finally asked outright if I could come to her house. My husband laughed hysterically when her answer was, "Well, I didn't invite you to the house because I didn't have time to clean my *whole* house." She explained her family was leaving for Hawaii in two days and so she had items laid out for packing. I remembered her being the neatnik. She assured me I was mistaken.

I know I walk around the house straightening the pictures on the walls. The kitchen must be cleaned before bed, I cannot cook with a dirty counter, and I cook meat using the sterile techniques I learned in nursing school. I have, on occasion, cleaned a cousin's dirty kitchen in the early morning so that I could cook breakfast.

My brother still teases me about the train in my son's room. It is up on a high display shelf. When we first moved into our home I was positioning the train so that it would look good from the doorway. I made him move it this way and then that way until it was just exactly in the right place. He found this terribly amusing because this whole exercise was over about one inch. Being the tease he is, my brother will visit and deliberately leave his clothing on the floor. After about three days of visit, I can no longer cope with the "guest room." I will swoop in and pick up. Upon completion he will dramatically toss something down on the floor and dare me to leave it. I have yet to be able to take the dare!

Now, I am sure that there are many people that would find these characteristics a problem. I don't. As a matter of fact I like them. I like a clean and orderly house. When I have been unable to clean the house myself, I have been fortunate enough to be able to afford the help to get it cleaned to my satisfaction. Perhaps if I couldn't and wasn't able, it would become a problem.

When I spend time around friends that are very symptomatic, *oh my!* I recently spent quite a bit of time with a very good friend that suffers from coprolalia. I found myself "reporting" his use of some pretty colorful expletives. See...I still don't "use" profanity. "Reporting" other people's profanity doesn't count...it's not mine. I've stopped doing that now and have gone back to my usual modus operandi of mental coprolalia.

I have now added finger drumming to my repertoire. Drumming in the air will do, but usually on this or that is best. My toes go most of the time now. This is no small feat in my size 9AAAAs. There's not a lot of room for movement in there. I also wiggle my right ankle regularly. In addition to the old leg jiggles, I now shake both heels. I also echo many other tappers I see. The beauty of all of this is that no one ever notices. I do it mostly in the car or when I'm alone. Many of my friends are flabbergasted when I say I tic. It should be of no surprise to many Touretters that many of my doctor friends would deny it is possible that I actually have TS.

In conclusion, there is no difference between TS and who I am. They/we are "of one another," and that's just fine. I have just "another way of being," and wouldn't life be boring if we all did it the same way?

■ ■ ■

Please visit the Tourette Spectrum Disorder Association's Web site at **www.tourettesyndrome.org.** *There you will find other articles that Colleen has written.*

If you would like to contact Colleen, her e-mail address is **wangci@earthlink.net.**

IGNORE THE TICS

Jonathan Gennick

The first reasonably clear memories I have of doing anything that could be construed as ticcing are from the first or second grade, so I'd say I was seven or eight years old.

My mother once asked my doctor about my tics, and his response (I believe) was something to the effect that I'd grow out of it. My childhood doctor never diagnosed me. The good part is that my parents realized I couldn't do anything about the blinking, so they ignored it.

I was 23 or 24 when I was diagnosed with Tourette syndrome (TS). It was nice to have a label for the problem, and to know that there was indeed a real problem underlying my tics.

I consider myself to have a mild case of TS. The doctor who diagnosed me prescribed Xanax *(Alprazolam)*, but he didn't think my case was severe enough to use other, more drastic, medications. I would take it prior to making a presentation to a group of people, or prior to engaging in any sort of group activity in a business setting where I felt concerned about ticcing. The drug helped somewhat, but as you might expect, it did not completely stop the tics. This doctor had another patient with TS, so he had experience treating the disorder and was sympathetic to my desire for medication. After a move, I went through a series of doctors who were skeptical of my having TS, including one who was openly hostile to the idea. That soured me a good deal on the idea of working with doctors, and I no longer take any medication.

My most prevalent tic is eye blinking. I occasionally sniff, but I'm usually able to suppress that tic. I seem to have allergy problems, and I'm not entirely convinced my sniffing can be blamed on TS. Occasionally I go through a head-twisting, shoulder-shrugging motion.

When I was in elementary school, perhaps fifth or sixth grade, I remember going through this symmetrical sniffing tic. It would go something like this: I would breathe in twice in quick succession, and then breathe out once. Then I would turn that around, breathe in once, and out twice. That's not likely the exact pattern—I don't remember clearly that far back—but the principle is the same. I've noticed over the years that in business situations, I sometimes tend to emulate mannerisms, and sometimes speech patterns, of other people. I've never had anyone remark about it, so it must not be enough to be noticeable.

My symptoms wax and wane, but I can't say exactly when. For example, one day one of the neighborhood kids (my son's friend) asked me if I had an eye problem, and whether I had seen a doctor. I explained to him that I couldn't help the blinking. The next day the same kid came over, and remarked: "You're not blinking today!" Well, he was right. For whatever reason, I was calmer, more relaxed, and my tics were coming at a slower rate. I have worked as a computer programmer, and have had people tell me that I tend to stop my blinking tic when concentrating on writing code. That was true for the most part and still is true. I tic less when in heavy concentration. I tic more when stressed or tired. At trade conferences, I'm often both stressed and tired at the same time, so just when

I wish I wasn't ticcing, I'm ticcing like crazy. This is especially annoying when I'm the one manning the booth.

For some reason that I can't fathom, washing dishes often causes me to have a great problem with eye-blinking tics. I experience the compelling need to rub my eyes a lot, which leads to soapy water getting in and around my eyes, which leads to more discomfort. This doesn't happen all the time, but it's occasionally bad enough that I have to throw down the dishtowel and leave the dishes to my wife. This isn't an excuse to get out of doing the dishes! In fact, I do manage to wash dishes on many occasions, and my first job was as a dishwasher in a Big Boy restaurant. Still, this problem does surface sometimes and it's frustrating.

My oldest daughter, who is now twelve years old, was diagnosed with TS when she was nine or ten. I wouldn't say her TS is severe, but her tics are often more noticeable in public than mine are. She's gone through the following tics: kicking, yelping, screaming, sudden stopping, spitting, breathing, and probably some others that I've missed. Fortunately, the really bad stuff doesn't seem to last for more than a week or two.

I can remember once when she had this yelling tic where every few minutes she would give out a short scream. Thankfully, that lasted only a couple of months before something else took its place. She's very insistent on doing whatever she wants to do, and I can remember sitting uncomfortably through dinner at a restaurant, with the other patrons all obviously wondering what was up with my daughter. I know a lot of people will disagree with me, but that night her tics were unusually bad, and I think she should have agreed to take the food home and eat rather than putting on such a public display. I also believe that if your tics are egregious enough, that you should do whatever you reasonably can to mitigate them. This includes such things as getting enough sleep, eating right, avoiding stress, etc. With my daughter, this has been a constant battle. Her lack of sleep leads to more stress and more tics.

My daughter responds well to medication (so well that I might even try some of what she is taking sometime); enough so that I believe TS will be nothing more than a minor annoyance throughout her life. My son, knock on wood, exhibits no symptoms.

My wife is very supportive. She married me, after all, knowing that I had tics. My kids don't know it any other way, so it's not an issue with them. My daughter occasionally gets frustrated and blames me for her TS problems. And she's right, they are my fault, but it still hurts a bit when she does that.

No one in my family that I know of has been diagnosed with TS. I have seen, however, some of what I believe to be mild tics in a couple of my aunts and uncles.

Fortunately, for the most part, my relatives ignored my tics as I was growing up. I'm sure it quickly became obvious to everyone that I wasn't going to stop my eye blinking, so even though they did not understand why I was blinking, they just kept quiet about it. One exception was an uncle who would occasionally lecture me on how I should stop. I had acne when I was a kid, and one tic was to touch my face (sometimes to scratch my nose). My uncle used to give me long lectures on how I was causing my acne by getting germs on my hands and then touching my face, and that if I stopped touching my face the acne would go away. I felt bad enough about the acne, but to be told that it was my fault really sucked. Fortunately, I read a lot, and I knew enough to be skeptical, so mostly I sat, nodded politely, and then went off and ignored his "advice."

When I was about eight years old, I went to a church school, and shared a ride with some neighbors who also went to the same school. I sniffed a lot at that time, and the neighbors, including their mother, thought I was simply being crude. In the beginning, they offered me tissues. Then they complained about my "snorting," and the mother demanded that I stop doing it. I can even recall times when the mother would hand me a tissue and demand that I blow my nose. It didn't help. Eventually, after a few months, my snorting tics waned.

Dating was a tough thing for me. I never dated in high school, and generally did not have any type of friendly relationship with girls. Things changed a bit in college, when I began to date. At a social level, people aren't (generally) going to come out and tell you that they don't want to be your friend because you blink a lot, or sniff occasionally. Still, I can often detect people distancing themselves from me because of my ticing. The worst part was that although I grew up with TS, I never knew what it was that was causing me to act the way that I did. My self-esteem was very poor, and I completely lacked confidence in any type of social situation.

I haven't had many problems at work. In today's lawsuit-happy environment, no manager or fellow employee is going to admit that anything they do is in any way related to my TS. For the most part, I'm very good technically, and that seems to trump TS. People may be put off somewhat by my TS, but when they see that I'm the programmer who is finding and fixing the bugs that stump other programmers, and solving clients' problems, they want me around anyway. On the flipside, I often don't feel like I fit in with coworkers. Many is the lunch to which I've not been invited. Sometimes I wonder if this could be related to TS, but it may all boil down to personality differences that have nothing whatsoever to do with TS. It's not like everyone avoids me either.

As for others' understanding of TS, the best thing people can do is to ignore the tics. If someone is talking to me in conversation, they should simply continue to talk. This is difficult for people to do, I know. I don't particularly mind if people ask why I do what I do. It's probably better that they ask and find out than to have them wondering what sort of nut case they are dealing with.

I have been asked if I would get rid of my TS if I could. To that I say yes, certainly I'd get rid of my TS. I'd love to eradicate the tics. And anyone who wouldn't needs to have his or her head examined. I'm always amazed at the people who say they are at one with their TS and wouldn't get rid of it if they could. TS means that your body is not functioning correctly. If you had a car that was firing on only five out of six cylinders, would you just leave it that way? No! You'd get it fixed. Likewise, if I could fix my TS, I would.

■ ■ ■

Please visit Jonathan's Web site at **www.gennick.com.** *You can also send him e-mail at* **jonathan@gennick.com.**

MY DEFINING MOMENT

Vernon Frazer

At age forty-eight I learned that I'd lived forty-two years with Tourette syndrome (TS). The diagnosis signaled the turning point of my life. If the two cases of Hodgkin's Disease I'd contracted by age twenty-five taught me about living my life fully, then TS explained my life to me in a way I'd thought inconceivable.

My wife's friend Dia, a nurse whose daughter has TS, informally diagnosed me in November of 1993. My mother was diagnosed with St. Vitus' Dance as a child, so I assumed I'd inherited a neurological abnormality. But I didn't think it was TS. The one description I'd read of the condition conjured images of a wild-haired hippie screaming curses from a straitjacket. I felt as though I already had two strikes against me: the emotional damage I'd suffered from my parents' bitter divorce and my years as a high-school scapegoat combined with my history of cancer. At the time Dia diagnosed me, I was struggling through my midlife crisis, which came on after I broke up my poetry band, whose fusion of poetry and jazz had constituted my most significant and fulfilling artistic achievement. Given my emotional vulnerability, TS looked like strike three.

Dia assured me it wasn't. She told me that many people

with TS experience nothing more than minor tics, such as eye blinking and throat clearing. Cursing was only one of a constellation of symptoms. She said that many people with TS possess special abilities, such as being able to multi-task more effectively than "normal" people. My ability to play bass while reciting my poetry and directing my band fit this description. So did my ability to work on several writing projects simultaneously. The stutter that made my high school years a living hell was a vocal tic, not a developmental stutter. Many teenagers with TS have experienced brutal ridicule just as I did in school. When Dia asked if I "evened things up" by touching something with each hand, I knew I had TS; I'd been evening things up since elementary school.

After decades of analysis and treatment by social workers, psychiatrists, clinical psychologists, and cancer specialists, why didn't one of them diagnose the condition? Dia explained that doctors rarely encountered it and patients with TS seldom showed their symptoms at their appointments.

Although she didn't think I needed medication, we talked about the available treatments. Haldol's *(Haloperidol)* side effect of social phobia would make me reluctant to go to my job, where I felt painfully out of character, and the possibility of tardive dyskinesia would only trade one set of tics for another. As a writer and musician, the side-effect of losing my creativity meant losing the most important part of me. After living forty-two years with the condition, I would rather twitch, swear, and be a creative person than a socially appropriate zombie.

Several days after Dia's informal diagnosis, I phoned a well-known child study center to schedule an appointment to obtain a formal one. The receptionist told me the staff was busy, but that someone would call me back. I phoned twice more, at two-week intervals, but never received a return call.

In mid-December, while waiting for the call, a respected

British record company offered to release a CD of my group, the Vernon Frazer Poetry Band. Then, after the hope of reviving the band lifted my spirits, the company arbitrarily withdrew its offer the following month. For the first time in my life, my depression grew out of control. A psychiatrist whose hypnotherapy sixteen years earlier had helped me overcome my lifelong anxiety about dating, prescribed Prozac *(Fluoxetine)* without warning me about its sexual side-effects. Although it diminished many of my Tourette-related symptoms, the unexpected impotence traumatized me. When I told him I thought I had TS, he asked, "What makes you think you have Tourette syndrome?" Doctors would ask that question again and again, always with a tone that seemed to question my intelligence.

After waiting six weeks for the child study center to return our call, my wife, Elaine, found a neurologist at a major health center. The neurologist asked me, "What makes you think you have Tourette syndrome?" in an accusatory tone that seemed to ask, "Who are you to be taking up my valuable time with such nonsense?" I acted out the symptoms I rarely displayed in doctors' offices, twitching my left shoulder even though I had no compulsion to do so and lacing my speech with obscenities. The neurologist tapped my knees with a hammer and conducted several other tests that confirmed the existence of my central nervous system. When she finished, she said, "You can go now."

"Do I have Tourette syndrome?" I asked.

"If you do, the treatment is as bad as the disease. I suggest you see a psychiatrist about your anger."

How could a neurologist dismiss my condition then tell me to get help for one of its symptoms? Why wouldn't the child study center return my phone calls? Hell yes, I was angry! To hell with all of them! I'd make my own way, just as I'd always done.

"I'll call them," Elaine said. She told the child study center that something was grossly wrong when a man who tried three times to schedule an important appointment couldn't even get a return call. The appointment was scheduled for March 18, 1994.

When the child study center asked, "What makes you think you have Tourette syndrome?" I told them what I'd learned. But my preliminary reading didn't prepare me for the questions they asked. I didn't know that thought-blocking was losing your train of thought or the words to express your thoughts. Once I knew what it was, I knew I had TS. I could solve a problem almost instantaneously, even visualizing my racing steps of logic, but couldn't find the words to explain what I knew. Probably many people underestimated my intelligence because of it. Whether I was right-handed or left-handed wasn't a simple question. I'm naturally right-handed, but somewhat ambidextrous. "Did I count things?" was the easiest question to answer. I counted everything, starting with my morning deodorant strokes.

The team determined that I had a moderate to severe case of TS. When we discussed medication, they recommended Catapres *(Clonidine),* a blood pressure medication that also reduced tics. I said I was willing to try it, but that I wanted my psychiatrist to administer it since he was treating me for depression. They asked if I wanted to stay to participate in some studies. I agreed.

While setting up the tests, one member of the diagnostic team explained that I was able to play bass and recite poetry at the same time because people with TS have cerebral hemispheres that are somewhat equal in size and dominance, whereas people without TS have one hemisphere that's larger and more dominant than the other. The doctor also told me preliminary studies indicated that people with TS performed complex tasks forty percent faster than the non-Tourettic control group. Now I knew why I finished my assignments well ahead of my co-workers.

When I left the child study center, the impact of naming the unnamable struck. For years I'd suspected that people held me to a double standard. My inability to obtain jobs or promotions; the invites to social events that I never received; the fact that I wasn't asked to participate in artistic collaborations—none of this was paranoia. It was a lifetime of shoddy treatment. As I started my Jetta, I said in a tone low and determined as an attack animal's growl, "This shit stops now!"

But it took time and effort to make it stop. The side effects of Catapres left me too sluggish to exercise. My cognitive abilities dulled so badly I felt as though I'd lost thirty points off my IQ. After my experience with antidepressants, I worried that Catapres was causing sexual side-effects as well. An off-night with Elaine prompted me to call the child study center.

"I'm not your doctor," the leader of the diagnostic team told me. "You should talk to your psychiatrist."

"He said he doesn't have much experience with Catapres. I'm calling you because you recommended the treatment."

"Well, how am I supposed to know! I only treat children!"

I needed a doctor who knew how to treat adults with TS. The team leader seemed unwilling to help me. Since my depression had left me too exhausted to fight my own battles, Elaine called him. "This man is trying to get help," she said, "and now that he's been diagnosed, everyone's abandoning him."

The next day, the team leader left a harried message on our answering machine listing several doctors in the area. A psycho-pharmacologist to whom he referred me wanted to put me on Haldol. I was adamant that I wouldn't take it. Several hours later he telephoned to tell me he'd spent two hours researching the effects of Haldol and understood why a person in the arts wouldn't want to take it. For the first time since Dia's informal diagnosis, I'd found a doctor who would listen to me. After my formal diagnosis I threw myself into learning about TS.

I read a popular reference book on TS, and it made me feel as though I'd inherited the bad seed. About halfway through, however, the book devoted one chapter to the positive aspects of TS. My creativity was a plus. My reflexes were a plus. So was my intelligence. (My other reading taught me that many people with TS score fifteen points higher on intelligence tests than people without TS.) The author listed symptoms I never would have associated with TS. Heat intolerance explained a lifetime of sweating profusely in temperatures above seventy degrees. Trichotillomania explained my continually twirling and pulling at my hair. Chewing my skin was another symptom. The deeper I got into the book, the more I felt I was receiving an explanation of my entire life, even though I disagreed with the author's conclusions. I had two-thirds of the symptoms he listed.

My first symptom appeared in the second grade, when I developed a short-term "paralysis" on the left side of my body. My mother and father took me to a doctor who prescribed a tranquilizer that tasted terrible and made me groggy. My stiffened mouth and gimpy left leg were typical first symptoms of TS. Within a few months I began my "nervous" cough and grinding my chin. Sometimes my parents told me to stop ticcing, but they never punished me for it.

When I was ten, my parents divorced and my TS became full-blown. Whether their vicious arguing exacerbated my symptoms or whether my symptoms made their fighting seem more severe had chicken-or-egg overtones. Either way, I think it played a role. I believe my mother's St. Vitus' Dance was actually TS that went into remission except for her thought-blocking, and that my father's genetic makeup contributed to my more severe case of TS.

The process of naming my condition sensitized me in other ways. When I read that it is common for people with TS to be shunned, it explained why I'd spent so much of my life without friends.

Near the end of the eighth grade certain students selected others for persecution. Somebody noticed my habit of going to the bathroom before each class, the result of a longstanding kidney problem combined with a Tourettic compulsion. A hall lined with students called out, "Hey P-P-P-Puddles!" whenever I walked from one class to another. I desperately hoped they would stop.

Instead, they continued. In ninth grade the students added the shout, "Your grandmother gives blow jobs to all the kids on the school bus!" Between classes, at least fifty kids made fun of my stutter and my bathroom habits, and called out obscenities about my grandmother. Some kids broke into my school locker, unwrapped my sandwiches, and placed toilet paper with catsup spots in the middle to create a bloody tampon effect. That winter my mother had to replace at least two winter coats that the students cut up in my locker. The teachers heard and saw what I was going through; I couldn't understand why none of them stopped it.

My mother complained to several parents. One parent said her son told her the kids teased me because they liked me. For the first time I understood the expression, *With friends like these, who needs enemies?* When nothing changed, my mother called the principal. He lectured the offending students in his office, but it just made the situation worse. By Christmas vacation of the tenth grade I thought I was getting an ulcer. I could hardly wait to turn sixteen so that I could quit school. I wished I had a machine gun so that I could kill every punk who ever made fun of me. My common sense told me a good student who never got into serious trouble shouldn't feel the way I did. I'd lived by the rules and the rules had failed me. I had to stop the abuse, regardless of how the school punished me.

The three kids sitting at the table behind me in Biology class had kicked my chair all year, causing my pen to scrawl across the notebook that I used for bonus points. I'd spent many evenings copying the pages their kicks had ruined. A few days after Christmas vacation they kicked my chair for the last time. I got up in the middle of class and bloodied one kid's nose. After class I told the principal, "You can suspend me if you want to."

"I told you to come to me about these matters!"

"I did. And it never did any good." I said, as I walked to my next class.

The kids called me "Tiger" for two days then they left me alone. That was all I wanted from them. I didn't want their friendship anymore.

Having to resort to violence because the people in authority wouldn't protect me caused me to lose all respect for the system. A month after the incident I discovered Jack Kerouac. His novels inspired me to become a writer, which would enable me to communicate without stuttering, and to live a bohemian lifestyle that rejected the mainstream values the teachers and bullies espoused. That reference book I mentioned earlier taught me that my choice of lifestyle was very typical of people with TS.

Moreover, the teachers didn't offer me the encouragement that might have kept me in the mainstream. My tenth-grade biology teacher once turned his back on me when my stutter stuck on a word in the middle of a question. At the end of the quarter, while penciling my third-quarter C on my report card, he told me I should be doing better. I suppressed my urge to tell him that turning your back on a student who's trying to ask a question isn't an effective motivational tool. Still, I tried harder. My fourth-quarter A raised my grade for the year to a B. In junior year, my American History teacher obviously respected the controversial stances I took in class discussions and my ability to defend them. He took me aside to tell me he thought I should be performing at an A-minus level instead of a C. I was flattered; he rarely gave As to anybody. I didn't make the A-minus, but my B the next quarter was closer to a B-plus. I responded when teachers recognized my ability, but I needed a lot of encouragement to offset the long-term damage my self-confidence had received during my parents' divorce and my early years in high school.

Although I gravitated to the bohemian culture, I can't say I received a much better reception there. For a number of years I was a denizen of jazz events in the area. At times I felt that people on the jazz scene didn't treat me as well as they treated other people, but I dismissed it as over-sensitivity on my part. About twelve years before my TS diagnosis, one of the regulars at our city's main jazz club started calling me *Twitch*. The second night he called me that name I confronted him. "Tell it to Bobby," he said. "That's what he calls you."

Bobby was one of the more intelligent and talented people on the local jazz scene. I'd never said anything about him that would justify his making fun of me. If he and his friends were calling me *Twitch* behind my back, probably a lot of other *friends* were doing it too. Years later, when my diagnosis gave me a name for my condition, my tolerance for them turned into contempt.

After my diagnosis I realized that many people I'd considered friends had dismissed my abilities before I ever had the chance to display them. Some of my close friends told me that people on the jazz scene tuned me out when my words rushed out in torrents; my rapid-fire expression of my racing thoughts disturbed them so greatly that they ignored the information I was trying to convey to them. A number of musicians I considered friends hired other writers for their mixed media projects. Only one person, the late saxophonist Thomas Chapin, accepted me for the person I am and included me as a poet on one of his recordings.

I was never able to land the part-time bookstore or record store jobs that would allow me to write without sacrificing many aspects of my personal life. For many years I applied for jobs only to be told, "We just hired someone yesterday." Looking back, I think the employers thought I was "too nervous" to do the jobs.

When I got social service jobs in my twenties, supervisors routinely called me into their office to say that I seemed nervous and to ask if I thought I could do the job, or to tell me that several of my coworkers wondered why someone like me was hired. Maybe I was supposed to feel grateful for the job. But the supervisors' point-blank assessments only increased my self-doubt. I felt so patronized and demoralized that I doubted anything I did would improve their opinions of my abilities. My relationships with the supervisors on my first two jobs after college became so strained that I resigned before I got fired. In both cases a number of my coworkers complained to management that I'd been scapegoated. Eventually, I had to keep a job or face a life on disability. On my last job, which I held for twenty-six years, several supervisors appreciated my ability to complete assignments quickly and accurately, but most of them considered my demeanor more important than the quality of my work. My diagnosis confirmed my gut feeling that I'd been a victim of continuing discrimination in the workplace. Many of the people I worked for would never reprimand a Latino or an African-American for fear of a civil rights suit. The week after my diagnosis, a supervisor tried to embarrass me in front of a representative from an important government agency. The next day I approached his supervisor and demanded a transfer. He told me I was over-reacting. I explained I had a medical condition that was protected under the Americans with Disabilities Act and could probably win a lawsuit over the issue. He arranged the transfer. I stayed on the job long enough to collect a civil service pension, and retired the first day I was eligible.

Considering that so many people never thought I'd be able to hold a job in the first place I'm proud of what I've accomplished, even though I never regarded the job as anything more than a way to support myself while writing.

If the social aspects of TS made my working life difficult, it made my love life virtually nonexistent. Since I never got invited to the junior high school parties where boys learned about girls, I didn't acquire the social skills needed to play the dating game until most of my peers were getting their first divorce. The few relationships I had were strained. The women I tried to treat well treated me badly. It took me several decades—and a good relationship—to realize that many women I'd dated didn't respect themselves enough to believe they deserved to be treated well. My lack of self-esteem made me wonder what was wrong with the few women who liked me. Hypnotherapy in my mid-thirties helped me control the intolerable anxiety that years of negative dating experiences had developed. When I look at most other couples now, I realize that Elaine and I are much happier in our marriage than they are in theirs.

My TS symptoms probably made me a poor prospect for women who wanted children. At the times in my life that I might have wanted children, I didn't have a partner. Moreover, my experience as a child from a broken home in the 1950s gave me serious reservations about having and raising children. After surviving two cases of Hodgkin's Disease I didn't want to risk passing it, and the accompanying social stigma, to my child. My TS diagnosis taught me that many of the factors that made me reluctant to have a child were actually related to my TS.

Even though I don't enjoy my sleep disorders, depression, or ticcing, I'd say that the most difficult part of TS is living with the social stigma that has cost me friends, lovers, jobs, and artistic opportunities. I've made some very good friends for whom my TS isn't an issue. Many acquaintances, however, invite me to social events as an afterthought. Other people look at me with pained expressions that make me wonder if my forehead reads, *I am you when your luck runs out*. People less intelligent than me treat me as though I'm stupid, then resent me when I prove I'm not. Even in the literary field I encounter social problems, although the quality of my writing has enabled me to overcome many of them.

Even so, I wouldn't get rid of my TS. Because of my diagnosis late in life, I've integrated my TS into my personality. The special abilities my TS has given me are my strengths: creativity, intelligence, speed, energy, and the ability to multi-task. If I could retain these attributes, I would consider not having TS.

Living with TS has taught me a tremendous amount about character and determination. Everything I've accomplished in my life has required overcoming intense opposition. Although many people laughed at my dream of becoming a writer, last year I had an opportunity to read in the *Established and Emerging Poets Series* at St. Mark's Poetry Project, one of the premier literary venues in the United States. My college friends—and many prospective employers—considered me too unstable to have a job, yet I managed not only to hold one, but to become one of the best in my field. I like to think that some of the women who turned me down or treated me badly occasionally have second thoughts.

I have never thought of myself as disabled. I still don't. I have a condition, not a disorder. My approaches to handling situations might be unorthodox, but they prove as effective as more conventional approaches. A childhood diagnosis would have made my mother shelter me. Nobody would have expected more from me than sitting home in a t-shirt, reading comics, and saying goofy things. I'm thankful that some part of me never yielded to the daily slaps in the face I've endured.

When I see parents agonizing over the future of their newly-diagnosed children, I want to tell them that TS isn't a curse. Most children with TS will live rewarding lives if their parents give them the love, respect, and support they need to survive the adversity of prejudice. I would tell parents to emphasize their children's positive attributes instead of punishing them for things they cannot help doing.

I probably would have accomplished the same things without a diagnosis. But learning that I had TS enabled me to answer many questions about my life that decades of introspection and self-analysis never explained. With the knowledge I gained, I developed the power to ensure my equality in the presence of others.

■ ■ ■

You can contact Vernon at **vfrazer@attbi.com.**

TOURETTE SYNDROME BY TRAUMA

Robert Jones*

Although Robert has reported that family members have symptoms of obsessive-compulsive disorder and attention deficit disorder, no one has ever been diagnosed with Tourette syndrome. Robert's story is a prime example of someone whose Tourette's manifested itself after a traumatic and life-changing event. This is not to say that a gene was not at work here; many times the genetic cause of Tourette's can lie dormant for generations, waiting for the right opportunity to show itself.

At age thirty-six, after the death of one of my sisters, I entered into a period of chronic atypical depression and a gradually increasing manifestation of obsessive-compulsive disorder (OCD). Around this time, my Tourette syndrome (TS) exposed itself first as vocalizations, then as jerking and sudden movements typical of "startle response."

I began seeing a psychotherapist around that time, and I noticed a marked increase in anger episodes. At the age of forty-one, I was officially diagnosed with OCD, and began taking the drug Paxil *(Paroxetine)*, at which time my TS

*An asterisk next to a contributor's name indicates that that contributor wishes to remain anonymous.

seemed to become more prominent. I must wonder if the increase in my Tourettic symptoms was not a synergistic effect caused by the large amounts of coffee that I was drinking to combat the severe sedating side-effects of the Paxil.

For me, TS typically appears as arm and leg jerking, usually when I have a traumatic or embarrassing memory, extreme stress, elation, or tiredness (usually late at night), and after ingesting too much caffeine. I will also occasionally vocalize—again when I'm tired—usually and thankfully I'm alone when that happens because it is usually an obscene or racial epithet.

The Paxil did help some OCD symptoms, but after a period of time some returned, just as severe as before. Yet, strangely enough, after discontinuing the Paxil, the OCD dramatically decreased. At least one other OCD sufferer I have spoken with has had similar experiences. I think there is a lot more research that needs to be done regarding the long-term effects of anti-depressants and serotonin agents. However, these Tourettic episodes still occur, usually in a private setting and with some degree of diminishment since I stopped taking the drugs last summer.

AFTERWORD

Four years ago my life took an unexpected turn when I was diagnosed with Tourette syndrome. Since that time, I have experienced many emotional highs and lows. But I have never experienced a more incredible feeling than having the opportunity to be involved in this project. *Getting Personal* is a coming together of souls; a merging of experiences. I never thought I would have the pleasure of meeting twenty-one other individuals who know exactly what I feel every minute of every day. As this book goes to publication, I reminisce on the past two years of my life. Working on this book has been an incredible journey. There was so much to tell: about myself, about others, and about this world of Tourette's in which we live. I hope you have enjoyed the journey as much as I have.

TOURETTE SYNDROME RESOURCES

There are simply too many resources to list in this publication. To avoid frustration with information that may be dated by the time you read this publication, I have chosen to list the major contact centers for information and support. Please contact these organizations for more additional information, resources, and a listing of the closest chapter or support group to you.

Tourette Syndrome Association (U.S.)
42-40 Bell Boulevard
Bayside NY 11361
Phone: 718-224-2999
Fax: 718-279-9596
E-mail: ts@tsa-usa.org
Web site: www.tsa-usa.org

Tourette Syndrome Foundation of Canada
206-194 Jarvis Street,
Toronto, ON M5B 2B7
Phone: 800-361-3120 (within Canada only) or 416-861-8398
Fax: 416-861-2472
E-mail: tsfc@tourette.ca
Web site: www.tourette.ca

Tourette Spectrum Disorder Association, Inc.
Web site: www.tourettesyndrome.org

Life's A Twitch!
32 Donlea Drive,
Toronto, Ontario, M4G 2M4
Phone: (416) 528.1538
Web site: www.lifesatwitch.com

Association for Comprehensive NeuroTherapy
P.O. Box 210848
Royal Palm Beach, FL 33421-0848
Phone: 561-798-0472
Fax: 561-798-9820
E-mail: acn@latitudes.org
Web site: www.latitudes.org

Tourette Syndrome Plus
Web site: www.tourettesyndrome.net

BIBLIOGRAPHY

I have obtained some of the information in this book from the following sources.

The Biological Psychology Web page of the Department of
    Psychology, California State University at Chico.
Encyclopedia.com.
The Tourette Syndrome Association Web site.
The Gale Encyclopedia of Childhood and Adolescence.
The Association of Comprehensive NeuroTherapy Web site.
Tourette Syndrome: The Facts by Mary M. Robertson, Simon
    Baron-Cohen (Oxford University Press) ISBN:
    019852398X.
Living With Tourette Syndrome by Elaine Fantle Shimberg,
    Introduction by Elaine Shapiro (Fireside) ISBN:
    068481160X.

SUGGESTED READING

A Cursing Brain? The Histories of Tourette Syndrome by Howard
I. Kushner (Harvard University Press) ISBN: 0674003861.
A Mind of Its Own: Tourette's Syndrome: A Story and a Guide by
Ruth Dowling Bruun, Bertel Bruun, Contributor (Oxford
University Press) ISBN: 0195065875.
*Children With Tourette Syndrome: A Parent's Guide (Special
Needs Collection)* Edited by Tracy Haerle, Jim Eisenreich
(Woodbine House) ISBN: 0933149441.
Coping With Tourette Syndrome and Tic Disorders by Barbara
Moe (Rosen Publishing Group) ISBN: 0823929760.
*Don't Think About Monkeys. Extraordinary Stories Written by
People with Tourette Syndrome* Edited by Adam Ward
Seligman and John S. Hilkevich (Hope Press) ISBN:
1878267337.
Gilles De La Tourette Syndrome; ASIN: 0890040575
Gilles De La Tourette Syndrome by Arthur K. Shapiro, Elaine
Shapiro, J. Gerald Young, Todd Feinberg ASIN:
0881673404.
Gilles De La Tourette Syndrome (Advances in Neurology; V. 35)
by Arnold J. and Chase, Thomas N. Friedhoff (Editor);
ASIN: 0890047618 .

God Made Me Special: Tourette Syndrome, My Personal Story by
Ryan C. Farrell (Raspberry Publications) ISBN:
1884825222.

*Handbook of Tourette's Syndrome and Related Tic and Behavioral
Disorders* by Roger Kurlan (Editor), Marcel Dekker;
ISBN: 0824787870.

*Kevin and Me: Tourette Syndrome and the Magic Power of Music
Therapy* by Patricia Heenan (Hope Press) ISBN:
1878267027.

Living With Tourette Syndrome by Elaine Fantle Shimberg,
Introduction by Elaine Shapiro (Fireside) ISBN:
068481160X.

*Medications for Attention Disorders (ADHD/ADD) and Related
Medical Problems (Tourette's syndrome, sleep apnea, seizure
disorders): A Comprehensive Handbook;* ASIN: 0929519116.

Out of the Darkness: A Promising Future for Tourette Syndrome
by Nancy Freeman; ASIN: 1878159135.

Passing for Normal: A Memoir of Compulsion by Amy S.
Wilensky; ASIN: 0767901851.

*Raising Joshua: One Mother's Story of the Challenges of Parenting
a Child With Tourette Syndrome* (Henry J Rholsson
Publishers) ISBN: 0965750167.

*Ryan: A Mother's Story of Her Hyperactive/Tourette Syndrome
Child* by Susan Hughes (Hope Press) ISBN: 1878267264.

Search for the Tourette Syndrome and Human Behavior Genes by
David E. Comings, MD (Hope Press) ISBN:
1878267418.

Taking Tourette Syndrome to School by Tira Krueger, Illustrated
by Tom Dineen (JayJo Books) ISBN: 1891383124.

*Teaching the Tiger A Handbook for Individuals Involved in the
Education of Students with Attention Deficit Disorders,
Tourette Syndrome or Obsessive-Compulsive Disorder* by
Marilyn P., Ph.D. Dornbush, Sheryl K. Pruitt (Hope
Press) ISBN: 1878267345.

Tics and Related Disorders (Clinical Neurology and Neurosurgery Monographs, Vol 7) by Andrew Lees; ASIN: 0443026777.

Tourette's Syndrome and Tic Disorders: Clinical Understanding and Treatment (Wiley Series in Child and Adolescent Mental Health) by Donald J. Cohen, Ruth D. Bruun, James F. Leckman (Editor); ASIN: 0471629243.

Tourette's Syndrome: Finding Answers and Getting Help (Patient-Centered Guides) by Mitzi Waltz (O'Reilly & Associates) ISBN: 0596500076.

Tourette's Syndrome: Tics, Obsessions, Compulsions: Development Psychopathology and Clinical Care by James F. Leckman, Donald J. Cohen (John Wiley & Sons) ISBN: 0471160377.

Tourette's Syndrome—Tics, Obsessions, Compulsions: Developmental Psychopathology and Clinical Care by James F. Leckman, Donald J. Cohen (John Wiley & Sons) ISBN: 0471113751.

Tourette Syndrome by Donald J., Md. Cohen (Editor), Joseph, Md. Jankovic (Editor), Chris Goetz (Lippincott Williams & Wilkins Publishers) ISBN: 0781724058.

Tourette Syndrome and Human Behavior by David Comings (Hope Press) ISBN: 1878267280.

Tourette Syndrome: Genetics, Neurobiology, and Treatment (Advances in Neurology, Vol 58) by Thomas N. Chase, Arnold J. Friedhoff, Edited by Donald J. Cohen (Raven Press) ISBN: 0881679224.

Tourette Syndrome: Index of Modern Authors & Subjects With Guide for Rapid Research by Jesse Stall Winograd (ABBE Publishers Association of Washington, DC) ISBN: 1559147520.

Tourette Syndrome: The Facts by Mary M. Robertson, Simon Baron-Cohen (Oxford University Press) ISBN: 019852398X.

Tourette Syndrome (Twenty-First Century Medical Library) by Marlene Targ Brill (Twenty First Century Books) ISBN: 0761321012.

Tourette Syndrome (Venture, Health and the Human Body) by Elaine Landau (Franklin Watts, Inc.) ISBN: 053111399X.

Twitch and Shout: A Touretter's Tale by Lowell Handler; ASIN: 0525942165.

Understanding Tourette Syndrome, Obsessive Compulsive Disorder and Related Problems: A Developmental and Catastrophe Theory Perspective by John Michael Berecz (Springer Publishing Co.) ISBN: 082617390X.

(The) Unwelcome Companion: An Insider's View of Tourette Syndrome by Rick Fowler (Silver Run Publications, Inc.) ISBN: 0964637693.

What Makes Ryan Tick: A Family's Triumph over Tourette Syndrome and Attention Deficiency Hyperactivity Disorder by Susan Hughes (Hope Press) ISBN: 1878267353.

Children's Books

Adam and the Magic Marble by Adam Buehrens (Hope Press) ISBN: 1878267302.

Hi, I'm Adam: A Child's Book About Tourette Syndrome by Adam Buehrens (Hope Press) ISBN: 1878267299.

Audio Books

Teenage Diaries: Josh in NYC, First Kiss by Josh Cutler (Author) audible.com; ISBN: B00005488E.

Teenage Diaries: Josh in NYC, Growing Up with Tourette's by Josh Cutler (Author) audible.com; ISBN: B000054889.

Fiction

Echolalia. An Adult's Story of Tourette Syndrome by Adam Ward Seligman (Hope Press) ISBN: 1878267310.

Icy Sparks by Gwyn Hyman Rubio (Viking Press) ISBN:
    067087311X.
Motherless Brooklyn by Jonathan Lethem (Vintage Books)
    ISBN: 0375724834.
Skull Session by Daniel Hecht; ASIN: 0670876615.
The Woody by Peter Lefcourt (Simon & Schuster) ISBN:
    0684853930.

GLOSSARY

Terms that were mentioned in the stories in this book are defined below.

Attention deficit disorder
Attention deficit disorder is a biological disorder involving inattentiveness and distractibility.

Attention deficit hyperactivity disorder
Attention deficit hyperactivity disorder is a biological disorder involving the symptoms of ADD compounded with hyperactivity and impulsivity.

Autism
Autism is a developmental disorder that affects social and communication skills. Symptoms include impaired social interaction, impaired verbal and nonverbal communication, and repetitive patterns of behavior.

Coprolalia
Coprolalia is the involuntary uttering or shouting of obscenities or socially inappropriate epithets, which are neither purposeful nor intentional.

Copropraxia
Copropraxia occurs when an individual involuntarily makes obscene or inappropriate gestures.

Dopamine
Dopamine is a neurotransmitter that controls movement.

Dysgraphia
Dysgraphia is a developmental writing disorder.

Echolalia
Echolalia is the imitation of other people's speech.

Echopraxia
Echopraxia is the imitation of other people's actions.

Neurotransmitter
Neurotransmitters are the chemicals that transport messages between nerve cells in the brain.

Norepinephrine
Norepinephrine is a neurotransmitter that controls heart rate and blood pressure

Obsessive-compulsive disorder
Obsessive-compulsive disorder is an anxiety disorder whose symptoms include obsessions or compulsions; having one or both is enough for a diagnosis. An obsession is a recurring or persistent thought that is intrusive or inappropriate. A compulsion is a repetitive behavior a person feels driven to perform.

Palilalia
Palilalia is the repeating of one's own last phrase, sentence, word, or syllable.

Palipraxia
Palipraxia is a repetitive action, as when an individual repeatedly flips a light switch on and off.

Panic-anxiety disorder
Panic-anxiety disorder involves unpredictable attacks of anxiety that can cause symptoms such as rapid heartbeat and shortness of breath.

Restless leg syndrome
Restless leg syndrome is a sleep disorder involving frequent movements of the legs.

Serotonin
Serotonin is a neurotransmitter that controls mood, hunger, aggressiveness, sleep, and is linked to obsessive-compulsive disorder.

Sleep apnea
Sleep apnea involves repeated, prolonged episodes of cessation of breathing during sleep. Sleep apnea can be caused by breathing obstructions or by problems with brain mechanisms.

St. Vitus' Dance
Also known as Sydenham chorea, this is a movement disorder that is associated with rheumatic fever.

Tardive dyskinesia
Tardive dyskinesia involves involuntary movements such as tongue lolling or facial grimacing caused by side effects of certain drugs, particularly antipsychotic medications. The condition may be reversible if recognized early by withdrawing the affected individual from the drug, but it may be permanent.

PUBLISHER'S NOTE

Second Chance Publishing wishes to express its deepest sympathies to all those whose lives were touched by the events of September 11, 2001.

In memory of all those who lost friends and family on that fateful day, Second Chance Publishing is donating a percentage of the sales of this book to the Betsy-Tacy Society's September 11th Children's Book Fund. Please visit the Betsy-Tacy Society's September 11th Children's Book Fund at **www.childrensbookfund.com** for more information about this wonderful organization.

Second Chance Publishing is also donating a percentage of the sales of this book to the Tourette Syndrome Association of Tennessee.

ABOUT THE AUTHOR

Michael G. DeFilippo attended DeVry Institute of Technology and has spent the last fourteen years writing user guides and help files for computer software and Web sites. He is a divorced father of a five-year-old boy and lives in Lebanon, Tennessee. This is his first book.